Occupational Therapy Approaches to Traumatic Brain Injury

The *Occupational Therapy in Health Care* series

- *The Changing Roles of Occupational Therapists in the 1980s*
- *Occupational Therapy Assessment as the Keystone to Treatment Planning*
- *Occupational Therapy and the Patient With Pain*
- *Occupational Therapy Strategies and Adaptations for Independent Daily Living*
- *The Roles of Occupational Therapists in Continuity of Care*
- *Private Practice in Occupational Therapy*
- *Occupational Therapy and Adolescents With Disability*
- *Work-Related Programs in Occupational Therapy*
- *Occupational Therapy for the Energy Deficient Patient*
- *Occupational Therapy for People With Eating Dysfunctions*
- *Computer Applications in Occupational Therapy*
- *Sociocultural Implications in Treatment Planning in Occupational Therapy*
- *Sensory Integrative Approaches in Occupational Therapy*
- *Hand Rehabilitation in Occupational Therapy*
- *The Occupational Therapy Manager's Survival Handbook*
- *Certified Occupational Therapy Assistants: Opportunities and Challenges*
- *Occupational Therapy: Program Development for Health Promotion and Preventive Services*
- *Health Promotion and Preventive Programs: Models of Occupational Therapy Practice*
- *Developmental Disabilities: A Handbook for Occupational Therapists*
- *Occupational Science: The Foundation for New Models of Practice*
- *Occupational Therapy Approaches to Traumatic Brain Injury*

Occupational Therapy Approaches to Traumatic Brain Injury

Jerry A. Johnson
Editor
Laura H. Krefting
Guest Editor

The Haworth Press
New York • London

Occupational Therapy Approaches to Traumatic Brain Injury has also been published as *Occupational Therapy in Health Care*, Volume 7, Number 1 1990.

The Haworth Press, Inc., 10 Alice Street, Binghamton, NY 13904-1580
EUROSPAN/Haworth, 3 Henrietta Street, London WC2E 8LU England

Library of Congress Cataloging-in-Publication Data

Occupational therapy approaches to traumatic brain injury / Jerry A. Johnson, editor; Laura H. Krefting, guest editor.

p. cm.

"Has also been published as Occupational therapy in health care, volume 7, number 1, 1990"—T.p. verso.

Includes bibliographical references.

ISBN 1-56024-064-4 (alk. paper)

1. Brain—Wounds and injuries—Patients—Rehabilitation. 2. Occupational therapy. 3. Brain—Wounds and injuries—Patients—Family relationships. I. Johnson, Jerry A. II. Krefting, Laura H.

[DNLM: 1. Brain Injuries—psychology. 2. Brain Injuries—rehabilitation. 3. Family. 4. Occupational Therapy—psychology. W1 OC601H v. 7 no. 1 / WL 354 015]

RD594.027 1990
617.4'81044—dc20
DNLM
for Library of Congress

90-5178
CIP

Occupational Therapy Approaches to Traumatic Brain Injury

CONTENTS

BOOK REVIEW

ABOUT THE EDITORS

Jerry A. Johnson, MBA, EdD, OTR, FAOTA, is President of Context, Inc., and Editor of *Occupational Therapy in Health Care*. She was Founder, Professor, and Director of the Occupational Therapy Department at Boston University (1963-1971), and more recently was Professor and Elias Michael Director of Occupational Therapy at Washington University in St. Louis. She served as President of the American Occupational Therapy Association for over five years and is a recipient of both The Eleanor Clarke Slagle Lectureship and the Award of Merit, AOTA's two highest awards. She serves as a national and international lecturer and consultant.

Laura H. Krefting, PhD, OT(C), is currently Career Scientist in Community Based Rehabilitation at Queen's University, Kingston, Ontario, where she brings a combined rehabilitation and anthropological perspective to her research with brain injured persons and their families living in the community. Previously, she was Assistant Professor/Coordinator of Graduate Studies in the Department of Occupational Therapy at the University of Alberta. Her area of research interest is community based rehabilitation. Dr. Krefting received her PhD in Rehabilitation and Anthropology from the University of Arizona.

Occupational Therapy Approaches to Traumatic Brain Injury

Preface

The impetus for this edition of Occupational Therapy in Health Care can be attributed to practitioners' need to discover what their colleagues are achieving in this burgeoning field. As many of the contributors have noted, this area of rehabilitation is rapidly expanding and occupational therapists are increasingly involved in the care of brain injured persons and their families. The purpose of this issue was to compile in a single volume a description of some of the ways that occupational therapists are involved in assessment and intervention from coma to community in order to illustrate the richness and diversity of this area of practice.

The area is an exciting one for a number of reasons. First, it is one of the areas in rehabilitation where there is the potential for true interdisciplinary work. Occupational and physical therapists work closely with speech therapists, nurses, neuropsychologists, vocational counsellors, recreation therapists, and a variety of physicians at different stages in the recovery process. The papers by Zweber and Malec and Dutil, Forget, Vanier and Gaudreault illustrate the fruitfulness of collaborative efforts. DePoy speaks to the issue directly in advising therapists to make use of assessment data from other team members rather than regathering information. Experience in brain injury rehabilitation more than any other field of practice demonstrates that the mixing of disciplines produces a highly effective and comprehensive treatment approach.

Another challenging feature of brain trauma rehabilitation is the need for long term intervention for both the disabled person and their family members. Although active treatment frequently occurs for one or two years post injury and even longer depending on financial resources and the individual's constellation of residual deficits, services are still short sighted. Studies are now documenting the need for lifelong services to maintain skills and to address new problems that arise long after treatment has stopped. Lifelong recovery is emphasized in De Poy's article describing the model of Traumatic Brain Injury Intervention. Moreover, there is a critical need for monitoring people with significant residual problems over their lifetime. The idea of lifelong recovery is double edged. It promises that progress is always possible but that residual deficits will linger, often for the person's lifetime. This aspect of brain injury also presents a challenge to the therapist in terms of working with health service planners to design programs that provide long term intervention and monitoring.

The idea of long term intervention and lifelong recovery suggests the importance of the lifespan development approach to traumatic brain injury. Although a brain injured person's functional ability tends to stabilize or plateau after a prolonged period of rehabilitation the effect of aging on functional status is now becoming an area of concern. This lifespan perspective also extends to the informal or family caregivers. The demands of caring for a brain injured family member or aging caregiver are now being documented and the idea of families requiring more or different types of services over a number of years is critical.

The principle that the family and disabled person are partners in the rehabilitation process reflects a long held principle of occupational therapy. As Dutil and colleagues, Painter, and I each point out in this volume, family members are as important as the injured person in the rehabilitation process. Not only does the family suffer devastating problems as a direct result of the injury, but it represents one of the major influences in the long term outcome for the disabled person. Too often family members are considered recipients of therapy; they also need to be seen from a health promotion perspective in terms of their long term influence on the disabled person when he or she returns to the community. A responsive family caregiver can provide stability as well as social and emotional support unlike that available from peers or from health care professionals. Based on this fact, efforts need to be directed at keeping family caregivers as healthy as possible. Health/morbidity studies on the burden of caregiver need to be conducted to underscore the necessity of preserving these valuable human resources.

The articles in this volume illustrate the heterogeneity of the patient/client group therapists label as brain injured. In general, professionals group traumatically brain injured persons together and distinguish them as a group from other disability types such as persons with spinal cord injury or multiple sclerosis. This "lumping together" of brain injured persons masks the complexity and diversity of functional problems exhibited and frustrates attempts at a "standard approach" to their care.

The diversity of functional problems is reflected in the need for comprehensive assessment. The articles by Katz, Hefner, and Reuben; Zweber and Malec; and Dutil et al., suggest the variety of assessment approaches available. Importantly, De Poy, Maley and Stanraugh and Dutil and colleagues focus on executive function, one component of cognitive processing that is often ignored in assessment and treatment.

In addition to illustrating a range of assessment approaches, the articles also present a variety of methods of studying traumatic brain injury. De Poy and colleagues and Katz et al. make use of the case study to illustrate their findings. My article is a descriptive work that arose from ethnographic research and Jongbloed and Morgan use the familiar descriptive interview. These qualitative methodologies suggest the emerging nature of the field of rehabilitation after traumatic brain injury and the need to build on the knowledge base by comparative and descriptive studies as well as single subject design and clinical trials.

This volume represents a sampling of the innovative work that occupational therapists are doing in brain injury rehabilitation. Hopefully, it will stimulate further growth in this area of practice.

Laura Harvey Krefting

Introduction

Jerry A. Johnson

This work contains an interesting variety of articles about the treatment of individuals with brain injuries, many of which emphasize the importance of the psychological and social aspects of treatment. There is also an important emphasis upon concern for families of brain injured individuals and their roles in and contribution to the treatment of family members with brain injuries, beginning at the time the individual incurs the injury to provision of care and support long after therapy is reduced or terminated. Finally, interesting and yet disturbing questions, which deserve attention and must be addressed by occupational therapists, are raised about patient perceptions and interpretations of occupational therapy services.

Readers, particularly occupational therapists, who review the contents of this volume from the perspective of patients or persons who are not familiar with occupational therapy may find that it raises valuable questions about the definition and description of occupational therapy services. The importance of considering the whole person, the biopsychosocial make-up of the individual with brain injuries, within the context of the individual's family and ongoing life "after therapy" is clearly identified as an important part of occupational therapy treatment.

However, in fulfilling these responsibilities, occupational therapists are confronted with providing competent services for the individual's cognitive and physical deficits and effectively addressing the emotional and social needs of both the patient and his or her family members. Consequently, academicians are responsible for insuring that students (both undergraduate and graduate) acquire knowledge and skills to deal with emotional and social issues of both the patient and family while also designing treatments that reduce physical and cognitive deficits, all of which must occur almost simultaneously. Clinicians must also evaluate psychosocial deficits so that they are justifiably included in the treatment objectives and provided during treatment.

This is a demanding challenge in health care systems which now require extensive documentation but also very efficient care. These pressures may result in neglect of emotional or social concerns which appear to have less relevance or to be less defensible yet ultimately, over a long-term period, may be the most important aspects of the occupational therapy treatment program.

In summary, this volume emphasizes and reinforces in very practical, meaningful ways, the importance of values long-held by members of the occupational therapy profession but often neglected in the demand for efficient, short-term services or under the guise that other disciplines will address such issues. In reality, psychosocial issues should be addressed when they arise during occupational therapy, and therapists should be prepared by their educational backgrounds and subsequent clinical experience to integrate them into the ongoing treatment program. Only then can we, as occupational therapists, substantiate our claim that we treat "the whole person."

Development of the ADL Profile: An Evaluation for Adults with Severe Head Injury

Elisabeth Dutil, MSc, OT
Andrée Forget, DSc, OT(C)
Marie Vanier, PhD
Céline Gaudreault, BSc, OT

SUMMARY. This article presents a new instrument, the ADL Profile, which is designed specifically for the head injured adult. The instrument is based on the model of occupational performance and on Luria's model of cerebral and motor functioning. It divides the concept of activities of daily living (ADL) into 3 dimensions: personal environment, home environment and community environment. It further delineates a number of activities, tasks and operations under each of these dimensions. The article presents a rationale for the instrument's development, a description of the development process and the preliminary validation work, and details of the instrument itself.

Elisabeth Dutil is Associate Professor, Andrée Forget is Professor and Marie Vanier is Assistant Professor of Research at the School of Rehabilitation, University of Montreal. Céline Gaudreault is Research Assistant. All authors are associated with the Research Centre of the Rehabilitation Institute of Montreal. This project is being jointly funded by the "Fonds de la Recherche en Santé du Québec" and the "Régie d'Assurance Automobile du Québec."

Acknowledgements: We wish to express our gratitude to the patients and their families who are participating in this study. We also thank Brigitte Lamarre and Caroline Gingras who worked as research assistants, Josée Labelle, José Maurice and Jacinthe Valiquette from the Occupational Therapy Department of the Rehabilitation Institute of Montréal, Louise Vézina, Occupational Therapist at the Hopital du Sacré-Coeur as well as Michelle Dell'Aniello and Pierre-Yves Therriault, graduate students, for their work on this project. Finally, we want to extend our appreciation to Rhoda Weiss-Lambrou for her editing comments.

INTRODUCTION

The rehabilitation of severely head injured people presents a special challenge due to the variety of physical and psychological changes that affect these patients. As the large majority are young adults, the most important long-term objective of their rehabilitation program is return to previous social and vocational activities (Najenson et al., 1974).

Following severe traumatic head injury, physical and psychological changes may be numerous and varied. At the physical level, the main deficits are related to muscle tone, mobility, coordination, balance, endurance and speed (Jennett and Teasdale, 1981). The major disturbances are, however, psychological in nature (Najenson et al., 1974; Brooks, Campsie, Symington, Beattie and McKinlay, 1986). Among these, deficits in speed of mental processes, attention, memory, learning and reasoning are the most prevalent (Brooks, 1984). Other deficits are also frequent including: irritability, lack of motivation, apathy and problems in regulating behavior (desinhibition) and mood (Brooks et al., 1986; Mazaux, 1986).

In addition, Lezak (1982) has stressed the importance of difficulties with executive functions which are defined as the mental capacities necessary for formulating goals, planning how to achieve them and performing them in an effective manner. All of these deficits have a negative impact on autonomy in relation to the execution of activities of daily living (ADL).

According to Brown (1988), no published research has specifically studied the influence of the psychological deficits seen in adults who sustained a severe head injury on performance of functional living skills. She defined functional living skills as "those skills (other than basic self-care skills) requiring higher level cognitive processing in order to perform." (p. 9) She reported, however, that studies on persons with mental retardation or Alzheimer's disease have suggested that there is a relationship between intellectual and/or cognitive ability and functional performance.

As independence in ADL is generally considered a prerequisite to successful social and vocational reintegration (Reed, 1984), it is important to carefully assess these skills in order to better understand the impact of the injury and to devise appropriate rehabilitation programs. The purpose of this study was to develop an ADL evaluation instrument for head injured adults. This paper will firstly review existing ADL tools and will then present a rationale for the development of the ADL Profile. This instrument will be described in terms of its design, procedures and scoring system. The paper concludes with recommendations for future studies.

A REVIEW OF ADL EVALUATIONS

A number of common ADL assessment instruments were reviewed for their relevance to the head injured population. Five criteria were used to evaluate these instruments: (1) underlying conceptual model; (2) pertinence of variables; (3) assessment method; (4) psychometric qualities; and (5) scoring system. These criteria were considered to be minimum requirements for an assessment instrument. The following presents a summary of this analysis.

Underlying Conceptual Model

A well defined conceptual model demonstrates how concepts are developed, defined and organized into a coherent whole instead of being a simple reflection of an accumulation of information. The large majority of ADL evaluation tools do not clearly specify on which conceptual model they have been developed. Among those that do, is the Index of ADL (Katz, Ford, Moskowitz, Jackson and Jaffe, 1963) which is based on a model derived from concepts related to ontogenesis and anthropology. This tool was designed for the aged and the chronically ill. Its main assumptions are that the functions that are impaired earlier will recover first, and that the recovery sequence parallels normal child development and behavior of primitive societies. This developmental model was considered inappropriate in the case of adults who sustained a head injury, because these patients do not suffer from a disease in which impairments and disabilities are developing progressively but rather of the consequences of a sudden trauma.

The Rivermead ADL Assessment (Whitting and Lincoln, 1980)

was used with hemiplegic and head injured patients. It is based on a hierarchy model that follows the specific recovery pattern observed in hemiplegic patients. Tasks are evaluated according to a progression from simple to complex based mostly on their sensori-motor component which is not the most important aspect to consider for head injured patients (Najenson et al., 1974; Brooks et al., 1986).

Some tools such as the "Système de mesure d'autonomie fonctionnelle" (Hébert, Carrier and Bilodeau, 1988) and the Functional Independence Measure (Granger and Gresham, 1984) are based on the World Health Organization's model of impairment, disability and handicap (Organisation mondiale de la santé, 1984). They were considered but rejected due to the difficulty in reaching a consensus on the operational definition of the concepts on which this model is based, especially the concept of handicap (Fougeyrollas, Saint-Michel and Blouin, 1989).

Pertinence of Variables

An adequate conceptual basis for an ADL evaluation defines the scope of the instrument and the variables included in the instrument. Because no unified ADL model has been defined (Reed, 1984), there is no consensus on the variables which should be included in ADL assessments and on which items should be measured to evaluate these concepts.

One of the major limitations of existing instruments is that some tools assess tasks and functions as if they were at the same conceptual level; for instance, they include tasks such as taking a bath or putting on clothes with variables like memory, prehension, mobility or continence which are not tasks but cognitive, physical or physiological functions.

Another difficulty with the existing tools is the inconsistency in breath of the definition of ADL. In some tools, the concept of ADL is wide and includes items such as inter-personal skills and community resources. In widely used ADL assessments such as the Barthel Index (Mahoney and Barthel, 1965), the Katz Index of ADL (Katz et al., 1963) and the Kenny Self-Care Evaluation (Schoening and Iversen, 1968), the concept of ADL is limited to personal care activities such as feeding, bathing, toileting, dressing and transfers.

With a head injured population, the area of personal care is generally not the functional area most affected; the problems lie mostly with the more complex home and community activities (Brooks, McKinlay, Symington, Beattie and Campsie, 1987). An appropriate ADL tool should therefore include variables derived from a wide perspective of ADL.

Assessment Method

Autonomy in ADL can be assessed through direct observation of the person performing ADL tasks and through interviews or questionnaires to the patient and/or a significant other, usually a family member. Direct observation is made while the person performs a task in a natural or simulated environment; this method assesses what the patient can do. Although it may be more costly because it usually takes more time, direct observation was found to yield more appropriate information and allowed for a better understanding of the patient's difficulties than other assessment methods in a study conducted with intellectually deficient subjects (Klein-Parris, Clermont-Michel and O'Neill, 1986).

Self-administered questionnaires such as the Riverdale Skills Assessment (Brown, 1988) emphasize the assessment of what the patient actually does in his/her living environment. With severely head injured adults, however, this method often yields unreliable results because of the tendency for these persons to lack self-awareness and to over-estimate their abilities. Useful information such as the patient's perception of own abilities can, however, be derived from self-administered questionnaires, but they should be complemented by a questionnaire completed by a significant other living with the patient (McKinlay and Brooks, 1984). Questionnaires and/or interviews are most useful after the patient has left the hospital or rehabilitation centre as they will yield information on how the patient really manages in a natural environment and is not prompted to do a specific task. Because direct observation and questionnaires complement each other, it was decided to use a tool that included both assessment methods.

Psychometric Qualities

Few ADL tools have been submitted to rigorous testing of their psychometric properties such as reliability and validity. In addition, norms are usually not included in ADL assessments. A recently published article (Law and Letts, 1989) analyzed thirteen well-known ADL scales and revealed that although a few tools have demonstrated adequate reliability and validity (for example, the Katz Index of ADL, the Barthel Index and the Klein-Bell Assessment) they tend to focus on the personal care dimension of ADL. They were therefore found inappropriate to assess a wide range of ADL for the head injured adult.

No ADL instrument that included norms was found although Brown (1988) has done some work on norms with a small sample size (N = 50) on the Riverdale Skills Assessment. It can be argued that ADL can be performed by every healthy adult; consequently, norms are not necessary. While this is probably true for basic personal care activities, it may not be the case for the more complex home and community tasks.

Scoring System

Scores on ADL assessments are usually based on the degree of physical or mechanical (technical aid) assistance needed by the subject to perform a task, and often there is no difference in scoring between need for physical assistance and need for a technical aid. Tools that include need for verbal assistance are rare.

In addition, most ADL assessments emphasize the sensori-motor component of tasks and rarely consider the cognitive, behavioral and executive deficits that may impair performance such as lack of concentration, difficulties in planning, apathy, inertia and lack of motivation which often characterize the head injured adult. With these patients, criteria such as time, ability to plan and structure the activity, to initiate the task and to self-correct errors are important. These are rarely included except for time which is considered in some tools (Hébert et al., 1988: Mahoney et al., 1965). Another problem area that is lacking in most ADL scales is the lack of identification of specific causes of failure; this type of information would help to plan intervention strategies. In most cases, the scoring system of existing evaluation tools does not consider this parameter.

In conclusion, a review of the literature was done to select a tool to assess the performance of adults with severe head injury in ADL. Although there is a large number of published and unpublished ADL assessments, examination of these tools lead to identification of several problems, some general in nature and others more specifically related to application with a head injured population. No tool was found that met the five criteria which were identified to be essential: (1) have a well defined conceptual model applicable to the population under study; (2) assess variables that are pertinent for patients with head injury; (3) assess what the patient can do and what he actually does; (4) have good psychometric qualities, and (5) have a scoring system that supplies useful information for planning therapy and social and vocational reintegration. It was therefore found necessary to develop such a tool.

DEVELOPMENT OF THE ADL PROFILE

Selection of a Conceptual Model

The ADL Profile is the first component of an Occupational Profile which is based on the conceptual model of Occupational Performance (Reed, 1984). This model includes three major performance skills: ADL, leisure and work, and the following performance components: motor functioning, sensori-integrative functioning, psychological functioning, including cognitive functioning and social functioning. These components affect the person's ability to perform occupational tasks or performance skills (Reed, 1984). This article addresses only the ADL parameter of the Occupational Profile.

The organization of concepts of the ADL Profile was first based on an environmental continuum (Lawton, 1983) which led to the identification of three dimensions of ADL similar to the ones described by Wahlstrom (1983); these are related to self-care skills (personal environment), home skills (house environment) and community skills (community environment). These dimensions were then divided into activities, tasks and operations according to an ergonomic model described by Crochart (1987).

Activities represent the overall tasks carried out by an individual within one dimension. Tasks refer to the overall operations performed by a person under specified conditions, in a specific place and within a certain amount of time. Operations are the smallest functional unit that can be identified in the process of performing a task. This model was used to organize the variables to be assessed in a coherent manner. The model is presented in Figure 1.

Identification of Pertinent Variables

In order to select the items to be included in the ADL Profile, a list of 96 variables derived from existing ADL tools was developed. These variables were listed under the following categories: personal care, household activities, mobility/locomotion, use of equipment, communication and community skills.

This list was studied by eight occupational therapists involved

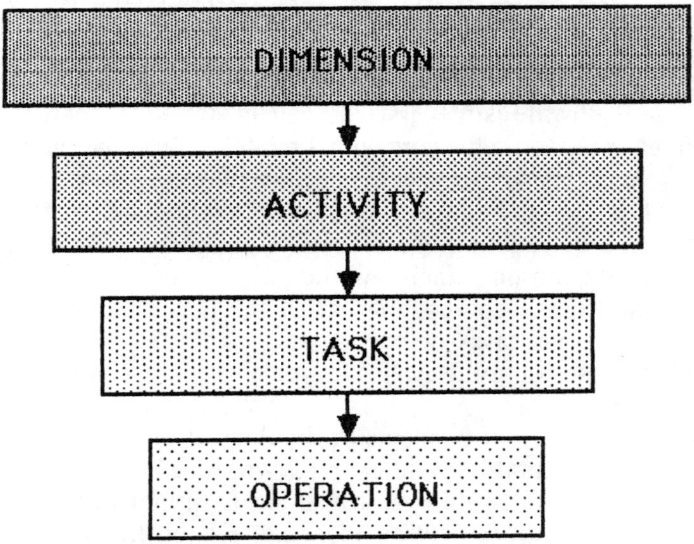

Figure 1. Model of the ADL Profile

with head injured adults through research or clinical work. These therapists were asked to determine if the item was an activity, a task, an operation or if it represented another concept, such as a function. They also had to decide whether the item was pertinent for a head injured population, whether any important item was missing and if there was a need to reassemble items.

This exercise was repeated twice and led to the identification of approximately 40 variables. Following further examination of these variables, other items were eliminated or combined and a list of 10 activities and 27 tasks was established under the three dimensions of personal care, home and community environments. This list was then discussed during a workshop attended by several occupational therapists, two physicians, a physiotherapist and a nurse experienced in research or intervention with head injured adults. These experts agreed with the proposed dimensions and activities but suggested elimination of one task and combining two tasks into one. This procedure resulted in the identification of the activities and tasks presented in Figure 2.

In the personal care dimension, four activities were selected: personal hygiene, dressing, feeding and health care. In the home environment dimension, two activities were retained: meal preparation and home management. In the community dimension, four activities were included: use of public services, transportation, financial management and time management. Appropriate tasks were then identified for each activity.

Operations were selected according to Luria's (1973) model of functional organization of the brain. This part of the ADL profile is still in the experimental stage and further refinement may be necessary. Luria's model describes three functional units organized in hierarchic order. The first one regulates tone and waking state or alertness; it has an important role in general disposition for learning and includes attention and vigilance. The second unit is for the reception, analysis and storage of information from the environment and is necessary for perception, praxis and language. The third unit (highest in the hierarchy) is for programming, regulating and verifying mental activity and is necessary for mood and behavior regulation and for executive and motor functions.

Lezak, who extensively described Luria's executive functions,

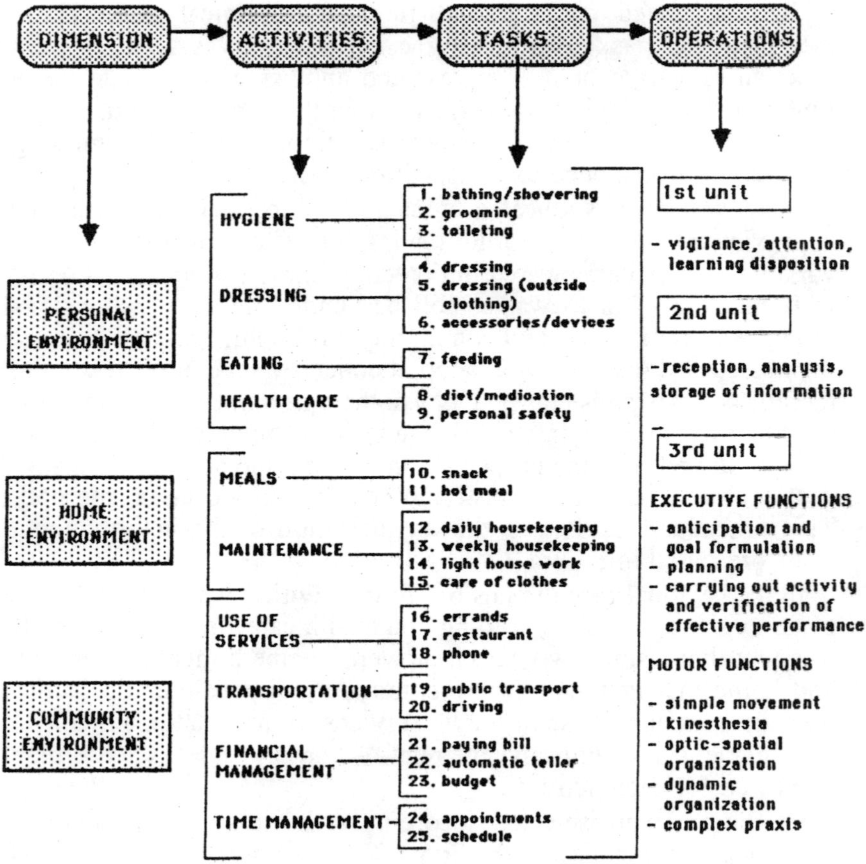

Figure 2. Dimensions, activities, tasks and operations in the ADL Profile

stated that impairment or loss of these functions "compromises a person's ability to maintain an independent, constructively self-serving, and socially productive life no matter how well he can see and hear, walk and talk, and perform tests" (Lezak, 1982, p.281). Her description of these functions is as follows (Lezak 1983).

1. Goal formulation refers to the process of determining what one needs or wants and conceptualizing some kind of future realization

of that need or want; it is bound up with motivation and with awareness of oneself in relation to one's surroundings.

2. Planning is the ability to identify and organize the steps and elements (skills, material, persons) necessary to achieve a goal. In order to plan, a person must be able to conceptualize change from present circumstances, deal objectively with himself/herself in relation to the environment, conceive alternatives, make choices and devise a structure and strategies to carry out this plan.

3. Execution of the plan of action is the ability to translate a plan into productive, self-serving activity; it requires the patient to initiate, maintain, and end sequences of complex behavior in an orderly and integrated manner.

4. Effective performance is the ability to monitor, self-correct and regulate the qualitative aspects of performance in order to ensure that all the elements of the task have been adequately performed according to the initial goal. Because it was found difficult to operationally distinguish sections (3) and (4) of Lezak's description, they are, at least temporarily, considered as one section in the present document (see figure 2).

Luria's motor functions have been described in more detail by Christensen (1984). The motor functions are: (a) simple movement whose basic requisites are muscle power and tone; (b) kinesthetic basis of movement implying intact kinesthetic afferent impulses to control the movement; (c) optic-spatial organization of the motor act which ensures the correct construction of movement in external space; (d) dynamic organization of the motor act which consists in the "conversion of individual motor impulses into consecutive kinetic melodies" (Luria, 1973 p. 179); and (e) complex forms of praxis or the ability to select movements that correspond to the overall plan.

Assessment Procedure

The first part of the ADL Profile is designed to assess what the subject can do. An assessment protocol which includes definition of terms, description of tasks and explanation of the scoring system was prepared and a preliminary version was pilot tested by one occupational therapist working in a general hospital and three occupational therapists working in a rehabilitation centre. A second version was then drawn up and is now being used in six acute care and rehabilitation settings in the Montreal area. With the exception of the tasks related to health care, the evaluation is done through observation of the subject actually performing the task in the institution or in the natural environment.

The assessment procedure is as follows. The head injured person is asked to perform a specific task and is given a minimum of structure. He/she must select the appropriate material and organize the task as well as the environment, if necessary. By observing the subject actually performing the task, the therapist notes the ability or inability to perform each operation of the task. The scoring system is described in the next section.

Scoring System

Each task is evaluated on a three-point ordinal scale according to the level of performance. When the patient is able to perform all the required operations with or without technical aids, he/she is said to be independent for this task and is given a score of 2. If the subject is unable to do any of the operations, a score of 0 is given which means that he/she is dependent for this task. When the subject is unable to successfully perform one or more operations, he/she is given a score of 1, which means he/she needs assistance.

When a task has not been evaluated, three mutually exclusive scores are possible: a score of 7 means that it is not pertinent to evaluate this task because of factors such as age, sex, or subject's habits, a score of 8 is given when the subject is not evaluated for reasons relating to self, such as mental or physical state or refusal to be evaluated; a score of 9 is given when the subject is not evaluated for external reasons such as missing equipment or inadequate environment. Figure 3 presents an example of the scoring system for the personal care dimension.

This scoring system is still being studied. The occupational therapists who are using the ADL Profile are generally satisfied with it; they feel, however, that in order to use it properly, they need a good understanding of the operational definitions of the concepts, partic-

OPERATION

Y	YES
N	NO
—	non applicable

		Vigilance, attention learning disposition	Reception, analysis storage of information	Anticipation and goal formulation	Planning	Carrying out and verification	Simple movement	Kinesthesia	Optic-spatial organization	Dynamic organization	Complex praxis
HYGIENE	1 completes personal hygiene □ sink □ bath □ shower										
	2 performs grooming □ teeth □ underarms □ shave □ nails □ hair										
	3 performs toileting (care of perineum, toilet use ...)										
DRESSING	4 puts on/remove indoor clothing and shoes										
	5 puts on/remove outdoor clothing and footwear										
	6 puts on/remove aids/ devices/ accessories										

Figure 3. **Example of the scoring system of the ADL Profile**

ularly those related to the operations. Further trial periods will determine if the system should be simplified or modified.

Reliability and Validity

Content validity was assessed through the selection of variables from existing ADL tools and the identification of pertinent items by experts as mentioned earlier. Preliminary inter-rater reliability studies were started through videotaping subjects being assessed and simultaneous scoring by eight occupational therapists. Each evaluator gave the same score to the subject but there was some disagreement on success or failure in some operations. Further studies are needed in this area.

Future Steps in Developing the ADL Profile

Studies on validity and reliability of the ADL Profile will be made through evaluation of a larger number of head injured adults. To establish construct validity, three factor analyses will be done using tasks as items and activities as concepts for each of the three dimensions. This will determine if all the tasks are relevant to the activity under which they have been classified and if the activities really describe the corresponding environment or dimension. Predictive validity will also be studied by correlating the results of the ADL Profile with psychological tests to determine whether some variables can predict successful social and vocational reinsertion.

In addition, two independent evaluators will be used to determine test-retest and inter-rater reliability; data will be analyzed using a single criterion analysis of variance. The importance of establishing norms for such a tool is presently under consideration.

Apart from these psychometric studies, the development of the second part of the ADL Profile to assess the tasks the head injured person actually does without prompting is presently under way. It consists of a questionnaire to the patient and a significant other living with the head injured person, and its objectives are to assess the changes in ADL performance since the injury and to verify whether the subject actually performs his/her daily activities when living in the community. This questionnaire includes questions relating to the 25 identified tasks of the first section of the ADL Profile. It is part of a larger tool that was devised by a group of researchers headed by Thomas Kay, PhD, from the Reasearch and Training Center on Head Trauma and Stroke of the New York University Medical Center. It was adapted and translated by our group with the authors' permission.

CONCLUSION

Following severe head injury, several problems have been identified that could affect autonomy in ADL. These patients should be assessed with adequate tools in order to increase the understanding of their abilities and disabilities in this area.

Although many ADL evaluation tools have been published, none was found to meet the five (5) criteria considered essential in the

ADL assessment of head injured persons. For this reason, the ADL Profile was developed. This tool is designed to examine, in a systematic way, the areas of performance that are usually most difficult for this particular population. When the second part of the ADL profile will be completed and more psychometric studies will have been done on the first part, it is hoped that this assessment will yield the pertinent information necessary to design better rehabilitation strategies. This should result in a more successful social and vocational reintegration for a greater number of these patients.

Those who wish to be part of the experimentation of the ADL Profile are invited to contact the first author at the School of Rehabilitation, University of Montreal, C.P. 6128, succ. A, Montreal, Canada H3C 3J7. The tool exists only in the French version for the time being but will be translated into English in the near future.

REFERENCES

Brooks, N. (1984). Cognitive deficits after head injury. In: N. Brooks (Ed.), *Closed Head Injury–Psychological, Social and Family Consequences.* Oxford: Oxford University Press.

Brooks, N., Campsie, L., Symington, C., Beattie, A. & McKinlay, W. (1986). The five year outcome of severe blunt head injury: a relative's view. *Journal of Neurology, Neurosurgery and Psychiatry, 49,* 764-770.

Brooks, N., McKinlay, W., Symington, C., Beattie, A. & Campsie, L. (1987). Return to work within the first seven years of severe head injury. *Brain Injury, 1,* 5-19.

Brown, H. (1988). The standardization of the Riverdale Hospital's home and community skills assessment. *Canadian Journal of Occupational Therapy, 55,* 9-14.

Christensen, A. L. (1984). *Luria's Neuropsychological Investigation.* Munksgaard, Denmark: Text and Manual.

Crochard, K. (1987). *Les activités du GESCOM en 1986.* [GESCOM activities in 1986]. Paris: Centre national d'études des télécommunications.

Fougeyrollas, P., Saint-Michel, G. & Blouin, M. (1989). Proposition d'une révision du 3e niveau de la CIDIH: le handicap. [Proposition for a revision of the 3rd level of the International Classification of Handicaps: the handicap]. *Réseau International CIDIH, 2* (1), 9-32.

Granger, C.V. & Gresham, G.E. (1984). *Functional assessment in rehabilitation medicine.* Baltimore MD: Williams & Wilkins.

Hébert, R., Carrier, R. & Bilodeau, A. A. (1988). Le système de mesure de l'autonomie fonctionnelle. [Measurement system of functional autonomy]. *Revue de Gériatrie, 23,* 161-167.

Jennett, B. & Teasdale, G. (1981). *Management of head injuries.* Philadelphia, PA: FA Davies.

Katz, S., Ford, A. B., Moskowitz, R. W., Jackson, B. A. & Jaffe, M. W. (1963). Studies of illness in the aged: The Index of ADL, measure of biological and psychosocial function. *Journal of the American Medical Association, 185*, 914-919.

Klein-Parris, C., Clermont-Michel, T. & O'Neill, J. (1986). Effectiveness and efficiency of criterion testing versus interviewing for collecting functional assessment information. *American Journal of Occupational Therapy, 40,* 486-491.

Law, M. & Letts, L. (1989). A critical review of scales of activities of daily living. *American Journal of Occupational Therapy, 43,* 522-528.

Lawton, P. (1983). Environment and other determinants of well-being in older people. *The Gerontologist, 23,* 349-357.

Lezak, M. D. (1982). The problem of assessing executive functions. *International Journal of Psychology, 17,* 281-297.

Lezak, M. D. (1983) *Neuropsychological Assessment*. (2nd ed) New York: Oxford University Press.

Luria, A.R. (1973). *The Working Brain–An Introduction to Neuropsychology.* New York: Basic Books.

Mahoney, F. I., & Barthel, D.W. (1965). Functional evaluation: the Barthel Index. *Maryland State Medical Journal, 14,* 61-65.

Mazaux, J. M. (1986). Réinsertion professionnelle des traumatisés crâniens graves. [Professional reinsertion of severe head injured persons]. *Réadaptation,* (no. 332) 3-9.

McKinlay, W. & Brooks, N. (1984). Methodological problems in assessing psycho-social recovery following severe head injury. *Journal of Clinical Psychology, 6,* 87-99.

Najenson, T., Mendelson, L., Schechter, I., David, C., Mintz, N. & Groswasser Z. (1974). Rehabilitation after severe head injury. *Scandinavian Journal of Rehabilitation Medicine, 6,* 5-14.

Organisation Mondiale de la Santé. (1984). *Classification internationale des handicaps: déficiences, incapacités et désavantages.* [International Classification of Handicaps: Disability, Impairment, Handicap]. Paris: Institut National de la Santé et de la Recherche Médicale.

Reed, K. L. (1984). *Models of Practice in Occupational Therapy.* Baltimore, MD: Williams & Wilkins.

Schoening, H. A. & Iversen, I. A. (1968). Numerical scoring of self-care status: a study of Kenny self-care evaluation. *American Journal of Physical Medicine and Rehabilitation, 49,* 221-229.

Wahlstrom, P. E. (1983). Occupational Therapy Evaluation. In M. Rosenthal, E. R. Griffith, M. R. Bond, & J. D. Miller (Eds.), *Rehabilitation of the head injured adult.* Philadelphia, PA: F.A.Davis.

Whitting, L. & Lincoln, N. (1980). An ADL assessment for stroke patients. *British Journal of Occupational Therapy, 43,* 44-45.

Measuring Clinical Change in Cognitive Rehabilitation of Patients with Brain Damage: Two Cases, Traumatic Brain Injury and Cerebral Vascular Accident

Noomi Katz, PhD, OTR
Dorit Hefner, OTR
Rachel Reuben, OTR

SUMMARY. The purpose of this article is to demonstrate the use of the Loewenstein Occupational Therapy Cognitive Assessment (LOTCA) as a measure of clinical change in the cognitive rehabilitation of brain damaged patients. Two cases are presented, one a traumatic brain injured (TBI) young male patient and the second an elderly male patient suffering from cerebral vascular accident (CVA). Evaluation and treatment combined sensory motor stimulation, cognitive remediation and functional approaches. Profiles of cognitive performance to follow-up progress during the process of recovery are presented. Recommendations are made to utilize occupational therapy ongoing assessments for documenting clinical change.

INTRODUCTION

Measuring recovery of function is one of the most difficult issues in the rehabilitation of brain damaged persons. According to Almli

---

Noomi Katz is Assistant Professor, School of Occupational Therapy, Hebrew University, Mount Scopus, PO Box 24026, Jerusalem 91240 Israel. Dorit Hefner and Rachel Reuben are affiliated with Loewenstein Rehabilitation Hospital, Raanana, Israel.

and Finger (1988) "Recovery is a theoretical construct that implies a complete regaining of identical functions that were lost or impaired after brain damage" (p.8). This definition of recovery, even though ideal, is very hard to measure because in most cases we have no objective measures of previous functional level of the brain damaged patient. Within cognitive rehabilitation it is assumed that most normal adults achieve a basic cognitive task performance. We, therefore, start by assessing the patients' *current* cognitive task performance. This assessment serves as a base line for measuring progress, and together with premorbid information, sensory motor evaluation and functional status evaluation in daily activities, is the basis for treatment planning.

The cognitive rehabilitation evaluation and intervention approach of occupational therapy at Loewenstein Rehabilitation Hospital (LRH) combines sensory motor, functional and cognitive retraining approaches (Siev, Freishtat & Zoltan, 1986; Zoltan & Ryckman, 1985), with differential emphasis depending on the individual patient's deficits and stage of illness. Treatment focuses generally on direct remediation of the specific cognitive impairments at the acute stage—phase one. While in phase two, when the patient is stabilized, work centers on compensation techniques in functional tasks. In both phases major emphasis is given to cognitive rehabilitation therapy in restoring function with direct retraining and/or compensating for impaired functions (Ylvisaker & Gobble, 1987). As Ylvisaker and Gobble state, cognitive rehabilitation has become the keystone of many rehabilitation programs.

Numerous treatment approaches are identified in the occupational therapy literature as separate entities, such as: sensory integration, transfer of training, functional and neurodevelopmental treatment (Siev et al., 1986); adaptive functional treatment approach or remedial treatment (Neistadt, 1988); behavioral approach (Fussey & Giles, 1988; Giles & Clark-Wilson, 1988); or deficit-specific approach versus information processing approach which defines treatment in a multicontext approach (Toglia, 1989). This appears to be theoretically sound, but clinically these approaches are not practiced in isolation. This is suggested also by the multiframe of reference approach in cognitive rehabilitation (Abreu, 1987; Abreu & Toglia, 1987).

In practice, a combination of approaches is used depending on the patient's impairments and phase of illness, premorbid capabilities and experiences, motivational and affective reactions, and environmental conditions. Cognitive rehabilitation may include only remedial table-top or computer training, or may be used in combination with direct activities of daily living (ADL) functional training, including also behavioral methods at certain phases of treatment. Work on sensory motor deficits using such neurodevelopmental concepts as body alignment, positioning and active movement patterns are used also to facilitate higher cortical function (Abreu & Toglia, 1987). Thus, Toglia's (1989) recent description of a multicontext approach which, as she states, shares some similarities with both remedial and functional treatment approaches, appears to be more fruitful clinically.

A vast research literature exists already about the efficacy of remedial and/or functional approaches but neither has unequivocally shown either functional carryover or generalization, and many researchers failed to examine essential variables significant to the outcomes studied (Neistadt, 1988). Nevertheless, the relationships between cognitive abilities and functional performance in activities of daily living and the effectiveness of cognitive rehabilitation has been demonstrated in various studies (Ben-Yishay & Diller, 1983; Bernspang, Viitanen & Eriksson, 1989; Carter, Howard & O'Neil, 1983; Carter, Oliveira, Duponte & Lynch, 1988; Soderback, 1988).

Based on the premise that cognitive abilities are significantly related to functional outcomes, the purpose of this article is to demonstrate the use of a cognitive assessment battery as one measure of clinical change in the treatment of brain damaged patients. Two cases are presented: one, a traumatic brain injured (TBI) patient, and the second, a patient suffering from cerebral vascular accident (CVA). Patients were treated by an interdisciplinary rehabilitative team and no claim of a specific occupational therapy treatment effectiveness is made here. Only the treatment process in occupational therapy is described, and changes in cognitive performance in conjunction with sensory motor and ADL tasks are followed.

INSTRUMENT

The Loewenstein Occupational Therapy Cognitive Assessment (LOTCA) was developed at Loewenstein Rehabilitation Hospital (LRH) in Israel, to assess basic cognitive abilities of brain injured patients (Katz, Itzkovich, Averbuch & Elazar, 1989; Najenson, Rahmani, Elazar & Averbuch, 1984). Basic cognitive abilities are defined as those "intellectual functions thought to be prerequisite for managing everyday encounters with the environment" (Najenson et al., 1984, p. 315). Cognition is conceived as a general term including attention, perception, thinking and memory.

The LOTCA battery was derived from clinical experience as well as from Luria's (neuropsychological) and Piaget's (developmental) theories and evaluation procedures (Golden, 1984; Inhelder & Piaget, 1964). The battery provides an initial profile of the cognitive abilities of the brain injured patient as a starting point for occupational therapy intervention, and a screening test for further assessment. It consists of 20 sub-tests and is divided into four areas: orientation; visual and spatial perception; visuomotor organization; and thinking operations. It takes 30 to 45 minutes to administer, and can be divided into shorter sessions if necessary. Procedures for evaluating patients with expressive language deficits are included.

The battery's measurement properties were established in various ways. Inter-rater reliability coefficients of .82 to .97 for the various sub-tests was determined, and an alpha coefficient of .85 and above for internal consistency of the 3 areas of perception, visuomotor organization and thinking operations were established using two patients groups and a normal control group (Katz et al., 1989). Validity in differentiating between known groups was determined with the Wilcoxon two sample test showing that all sub-tests differentiated at the .0001 level of significance between controls and each of the patient groups (TBI and CVA). Initial construct validity was examined using an exploratory factor analysis, which showed a three factor solution and a total amount of variance explained above 60% which is a substantial percentage supporting the assumed structure of the LOTCA (Katz et al., 1989). Criterion validity was examined within the CCI group for the visuomotor organization area using the Block Design sub-test of the WAIS (Wechsler,

1981). A Pearson correlation coefficient of r = .68 was found between the score on the Block Design and the mean score of the visuomotor organization sub-tests of the LOTCA, and a r = .77 when time was not measured on the Block Design. Almost identical results were found for a group of chronic schizophrenic adult inpatients (r = .69 and r = .78).

In addition, age level standards were determined testing 240 normal primary school children, 40 subjects in each age group between six to twelve years. Children's performance on the LOTCA were assessed to determine age norms of the various sub-tests, as well as to verify the hierarchical order of acquiring the various cognitive competencies included in the battery. Results show a clear developmental sequence in performance along the LOTCA sub-tests. Level of performance increased steadily with age, while the speed to perform the visuomotor tasks decreased concomitant with the increase towards maximal performance (Averbuch & Katz, 1989). These findings support the battery's assumed hierarchical order and the intended basic level of cognitive abilities measured with the LOTCA.

Thus, the measurement properties of the LOTCA were found to be reliable both in agreement between raters and in the internal consistency of its 3 component areas: perception, visuomotor organization, and thinking. The LOTCA was also found to be valid in differentiating between healthy adult persons and brain damaged patients. This finding, along with the results of a previous study where the performance profile of psychiatric patients was shown to differ from CCI patients (Averbuch & Katz, 1988), suggests that the LOTCA differentiates level of performance as well as enables differentiation between patterns of cognitive deficits related to the site of the brain lesions.

On the individual level the LOTCA is used at LRH as a measure of the patient's status over time, that is, as a measure for clinical change. In those cases in which deficits were present at initial assessment, the LOTCA is employed as a measure for follow-up on patients' progress. It is recommended that the assessment be repeated after an interval of at least two months to avoid simple memory carry over. However, learning as a possible explanation for higher scores must always be considered since many similar tasks are practiced during treatment. But it is precisely this learning, if generalized, that is the purpose of treatment, so that it should not be regarded as a threat to validity as defined in measurement theory.

TBI CASE STUDY

Jacob is a 24-year-old man with right hand dominance. He is Israeli born, unmarried, and finished tenth grade, spending the last two years in a technical junior high school focusing on carpentry. After three years of mandatory army service Jacob began studying for the matriculations exams as part of an adult education project. He was a truck driver when he was injured in a car accident.

Diagnosis

Cranio Cerebral Injury: Prolonged unawareness state; brain contusion; status/post left temporo-parietal acute subdural hematoma; status/post left temporo-parietal craniotomy.

Course of the disease: Jacob was injured on February 23, 1989, and hospitalized in coma. Brain catscan (CT) showed left subdural hematoma with slight deviation of the midline. A craniotomy was performed in the temporo-parietal area. After the surgery, while Jacob was still in a coma, a severe right hemiparesis was noted. Twenty days after injury Jacob opened his eyes for the first time and could perform simple tracking. Later, active movements on the left side began to return with an increase in spasticity on the right side.

Jacob was transferred to LRH one month after his injury. He was still restless, aware of his surroundings but had not yet vocalized. He was incontinent and was tube fed. Jacob was referred to the occupational therapy department immediately after his arrival.

Initial Occupational Therapy Evaluation

Three areas were evaluated: sensory motor functions, activities of daily living (ADL), and cognitive abilities. Communication abilities were assessed by a speech pathologist, and the patient was diagnosed as having expressive receptive aphasia.

Sensory motor function was evaluated based on the Bobath NDT approach which showed: no limitations in range of motion; right hemiparesis; increased flexor tone in right upper and lower extremities but no active movements; normal tone and active movements on the left side. Postural reaction noted were: limitations of equilibrium reactions in sitting but good control of head position. The patient used his left hand in performing various actions. Sensation could not be assessed because of his difficulties in language comprehension.

ADL evaluation showed that Jacob needed complete help in transfers, mobility, dressing and personal hygiene. He began to eat by himself using the left hand when the food was served and placed before him. He was still incontinent.

Cognitive assessment was performed using the LOTCA battery (see Figure 1). The evaluation combines observation of the patient's reactions, his task performance and manner of behavior.

General behavior during the assessment: Jacob collaborated, was alert but had a severe problem in auditory comprehension. He followed only very simple directions and these not systematically. He persevered in his spontaneous speech and it consisted of only two or three words which did not necessarily fit the topic.

Results of the LOTCA

Orientation: This is one of the areas tested using verbal questions, thus it was difficult to evaluate due to receptive aphasia. Through visual cues and gestures it was found that Jacob knew that he was in a hospital and understood the reason.

Perception (procedures for assessing aphasic patients were used): Visual perception at the level of object identification was normal using similar objects, but he could not name the objects. He had difficulty in shape identification and in identifying more complex objects. An additional problem was in identifying an object from partial information and performing an analysis of the input data, as in overlapping figures and in object constancy sub-tests, where objects are presented from unusual angles. There was no verbal comprehension of concepts related to spatial perception.

Praxis functions: Imitation of movements was normal but difficulties were noted in object manipulations and motor planning (ideational and ideomotor praxis).

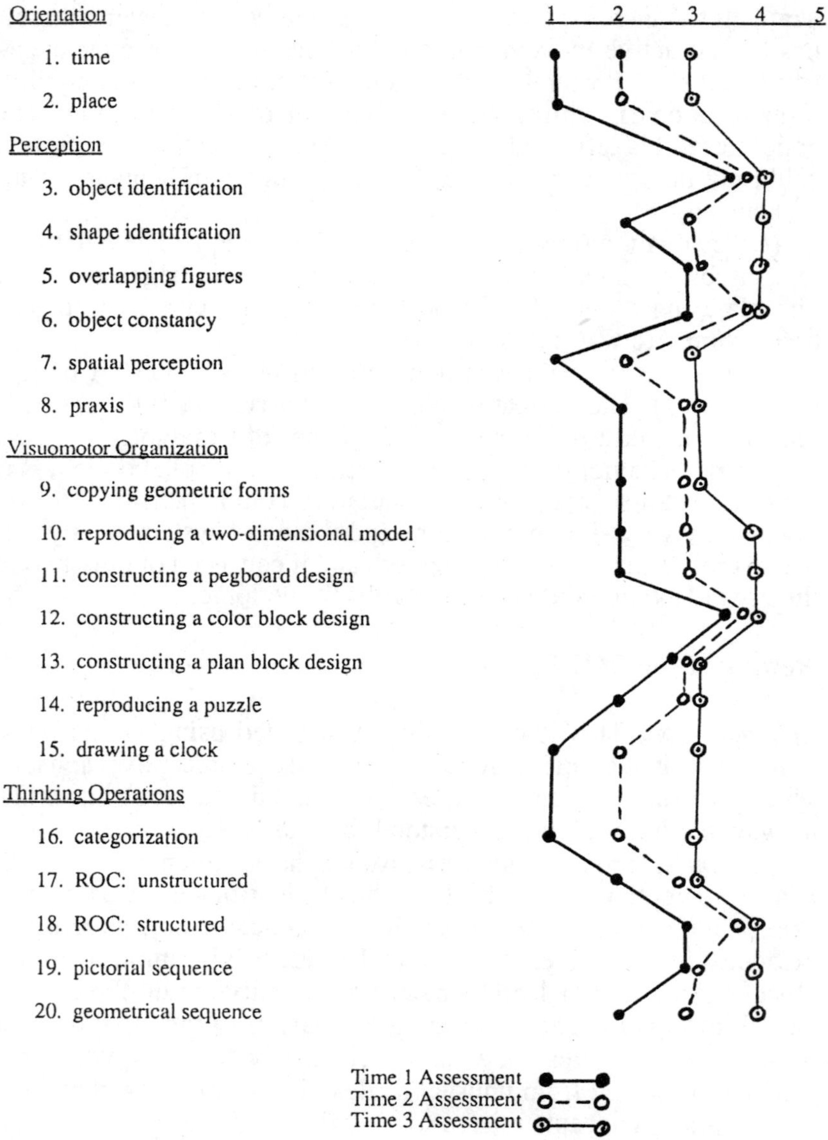

FIGURE 1. LOTCA Profile of TBI Patient for Three Assessments

Visuomotor organization: Jacob had problems in copying the basic geometric forms and could not copy the complex ones (difficulty in using his nondominent left hand may have interfered with his performance as he worked with his left hand only). He had problems in reproducing a two dimensional model, constructing a pegboard design and reproducing a puzzle, suggesting a problem in analysis and in comprehending spatial relations. Even though, surprisingly, performance of three dimensional construction was higher. In drawing a clock Jacob showed his understanding of the object but did not put in numbers the first time, in his second attempt he filled in 4 numbers (3;6;9;10) but the position of the 10 and the time 10:15 was wrong. Only by the third assessment, were numbers entered along with the right time but the organization was still not correct. (see Figure 2).

Thinking operations: Jacob was not able to group cards with drawn pictorial objects in any meaningful manner; he related only to colors when asked to group spontaneously geometric forms. When he was provided with a structured condition his performance improved. He performed the pictorial sequence correctly but was not able to verbalize the story, and in the geometrical sequence he could not solve the problem when he had to consider more than one criterion.

Attention and concentration: Jacob could attend only for a short period, and therefore the assessment was divided into two sessions. He had very slow reaction times, and his limitations in communication (comprehension and expression) contributed to his low scores.

Treatment Rationale Based on the Evaluation Conclusions

The comprehensive evaluation showed impairment in various areas but the dominant deficit was in language (aphasia) in combination with motor dysfunction and motor planning (apraxia). While the language impairment made it difficult for verbal communication, the impairments in motor planning and visual motor tasks made it difficult to communicate with Jacob in nonverbal ways.

For these reasons and because his basic visual perception seemed intact, the first goal of treatment was to strengthen the visual mode

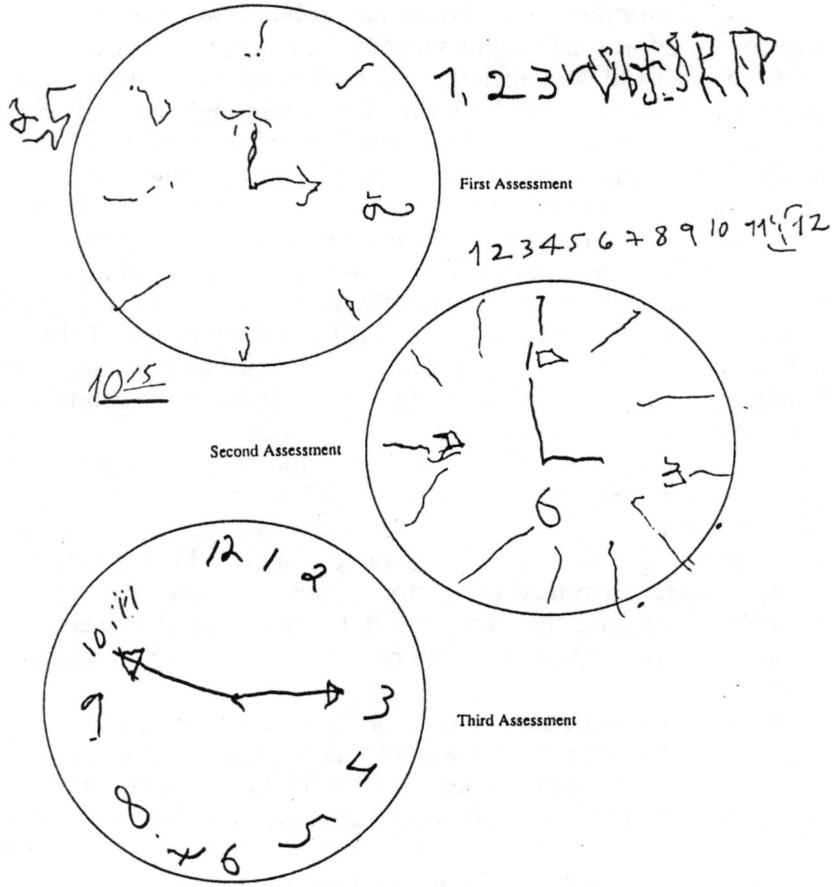

FIGURE 2. Example of Clock Drawings of TBI Patient

through cognitive training of visual tasks and only gradually introducing for training other aspects of impairment. Thus, the plan was to work with his healthy functional areas first and then to utilize these abilities to improve dysfunctional areas.

Treatment planning was based on the evaluation findings and on the basis of the understanding of the primary and accompanying secondary impairments. Luria (1973) states that brain trauma that causes a focused cortical lesion, resulting in a certain primary dysfunction, may bring about secondary impairments in all systems in which this lesion is involved. The fact that a focused cortical lesion may cause dysfunction of various cortical systems means that such a lesion may cause a whole syndrome as a result of the primary impairment. Treatment involves active participation of the patient, starting from the patient's level of ability and developing from simple to more complex tasks, providing initially detailed instructions and cues by the therapist and gradually reducing them until the patient is able to perform the task independently. Continuous and systematic feedback is an important part of the treatment process. "The aim of the training is to broaden the patient's capacity to handle information and transform it into purposeful actions" (Rahmani, 1982, p.45).

The Treatment Process

Jacob received individual treatment for about an hour daily, combining sensory stimulation, cognitive training and functional self care activities. In order to improve communication, parallel to the work of the speech pathologist, illustration with visual methods was used, and Jacob was encouraged to use signs and gestures. Starting with object identification and naming, the complexity of the objects was increased gradually to improve discrimination of items, part-whole differentiation, and identifying the most salient features in a situation.

An improvement occurred in understanding of visual cues, and this enabled training to improve orientation for place, using maps, and for time, utilizing a visual time table. In training to improve motor planning, which is fundamental for self care activities, Jacob was provided with a combination of experiences in ADL tasks, physical exercises, and table top constructional tasks which emphasized learning of strategies to analyze visual materials.

The focus in the thinking operational area was at first on reception of information, basic perception, and screening of a given input. The second focus was on processing of information by analyzing the input into its components and comparing it to other inputs, as well as learning concepts of classes and groups. The aim of this training was to teach Jacob methods of information processing, which would help him in decision making and problem solving. Jacob collaborated in his treatment with awareness of his difficulties.

Second Occupational Therapy Evaluation

After seven weeks in treatment, improvement in Jacob's condition was observed. To measure the changes, the same areas were reassessed. *Sensory motor* function showed improvement in fine motor left hand function, in eating, and graphomotor ability. There was improvement in posture and transfer of weight to both sides of the body and a return of movements in the flexor position in the right upper extremity. However, tone was still increased, and the hand was not functional. *In ADL*, Jacob became independent in eating, he could dress the upper body but not the lower body, he was able to propel a wheelchair by himself, he could control bladder and bowel, and he was independent at the toilet but needed help in his bathing.

Cognitive assessment showed improvement in almost all areas (see Figure 1). *Orientation:* He was oriented in the hospital's surroundings, functioned with an hourly schedule, used a watch and a weekly calender. *Perception* and *visuomotor* organization improved which is also demonstrable in ADL. Improvement was also seen in *thinking operations*, especially in the ability to categorize into concrete groups of objects according to their characteristics. In addition, there was improvement in auditory understanding and in spontaneous speech. He used more visual signs and gestures to communicate. Jacob's performance was still slow. The LOTCA took an hour but he had longer attention span than in the initial assessment.

Third Occupational Therapy Evaluation

After four months in treatment, a third evaluation was performed. Jacob was independent now in eating, dressing and bathing. He was still mobile only in a wheelchair but independent in its usage, and was able to transfer himself from one position to another. He was starting gait training. There was good recovery of function in the upper extremity and Jacob was beginning training in fine motor actions such as writing.

As his comprehension and speech improved, so has his understanding of the instructions of the LOTCA. However, he still needed visual demonstrations in more complex tasks. It is important to note that his expressive aphasia deficits improved more than the receptive ones which enabled a more accurate assessment of his orientation and abilities in sub-tests that require comprehension of verbal instructions. It can be seen in Figure 1 that additional improvement occurred but impairment still remained in areas requiring fine motor performance, verbal responses, and conceptualization.

At this writing Jacob continues to be in active treatment with an interdisciplinary rehabilitation team. His performance on primary impairments is still improving and he has not yet reached a plateau (Najenson et al., 1984). Once he stabilizes, the rehabilitation plan is for Jacob to return to live with his family. Prior to discharge Jacob will also undergo a more extensive neuropsychological assessment to further evaluate his cognitive abilities for possible recommendation for community re-entry. He will be referred to vocational training for a job in which he demonstrates an interest, and which utilizes visual skills and offers learning that is not primarily verbal in order to compensate for long term deficits.

In addition, Jacob will return for follow-up every six months as part of the follow-up program at LRH. At these follow-up sessions TBI patients are evaluated for their functional status at home and community, and if necessary, they are re-evaluated with the neuropsychological battery for cognitive abilities. The LOTCA usually is not used at this stage because the cognitive deficits most TBI patients still have are on a higher level. Occasionally this is not the case, and re-assessment with the LOTCA is performed to determine level of regression.

CVA CASE STUDY

David is a 64-year-old man with right hand dominance, married and father of two. He finished the eighth grade and worked as a driver until his stroke. He has suffered from high blood pressure for many years, has ischemic heart disease and a mild diabetes which was not treated. On May 2, 1989 David underwent a coronary bypass surgery. Twenty days later he suffered a stroke and was hospitalized.

Diagnosis

Cerebral vascular accident (CVA) left hemiplegia; left hemianopsia; status/post myocardial infarction hypertension. Ten days after his stroke, David was transferred to LRH. In a brain CT a low density area was found in the right occipito-temporal and another area in the thalamus and right capsula interna, which caused a wide right hemisphere damage to the occipito-temporal cortical area and subcortical thalamus and capsula interna areas.

Initial Occupational Therapy Evaluation

Sensory motor evaluation: Impaired equilibrium in sitting were noted. He tended to slip forward and to fall to the left side. Head and eyes were directed to the right, and he did not respond to auditory cues. Right upper and lower extremities functioned normally. In the left upper and lower extremities there was no limitation in passive range of motion, but there was no active movement. Hypotonia existed on the left side, and there was subluxation of left shoulder. Sensation on the right side was normal. On the left side, there was severe impairment in surface and deep sensation.

ADL evaluation: David was incontinent. He could not turn in bed or sit up independently. He needed help in all transfers, and in washing and grooming. He ate solid food only when it was cut and served within his intact right visual field, and he had problems with swallowing fluids. He also had dressing apraxia.

Cognitive evaluation: Administration of the LOTCA took several sessions because of a very short attention and concentration span which manifested itself in agitation, diffuse speech, and flights of association.

Orientation: David was oriented to place but not time.

Perception: He identified objects and shapes when they were presented in his right visual field. He did not differentiate among overlapping figures and had impaired object constancy. His visual scan-

scanning was severely impaired, and he ignored the left side. He identified directions on his body and relationships among objects but could not follow when changes in spatial position were introduced. Basic praxis functions were intact.

Visuomotor organization: David had severe problems in visuomotor organization with constructional apraxia. He was unable to perform any of the sub-tests in this area. See Figure 4 for an illustration of his drawing a clock, which clearly shows a left unilateral spatial neglect.

Thinking operations were not assessed due to insufficient attention span and concentration (see Figure 3 for the LOTCA profile). As a result of the cognitive deficits, David was also impaired in his ability to calculate; he could not read as a result of the impaired visual perception and unilateral neglect and could not organize himself in writing. David had awareness only of his motor impairment and ignored all other problems.

Treatment Process

David's primary deficits were left unilateral spatial neglect in conjunction with severe sensory motor deficits which caused a profound functional disability. Therefore, the initial treatment goals were: (1) to improve David's awareness of his left side of his body, and (2) to improve his awareness of his extra personal space. At this stage of treatment the auditory input mode was used since hearing is the most preserved sensation in patients with this kind of brain damage. David received daily individual treatment sessions of 15 minutes, which were gradually increased to 30-45 minutes. Sensory stimulation was given to his left side to improve awareness. At the same time there was emphasis on the symmetry of both sides of the body. To improve awareness of the external left space, treatment focused on tracking and turning to the left by providing auditory, visual and tactile stimulations. Treatment to improve awareness of both personal and extra personal space were combined through daily ADL activities of dressing (right positioning, right organization of clothing items, awareness of both parts of the body, and planning of the dressing process).

Gradually David's attention span increased which enabled treat-

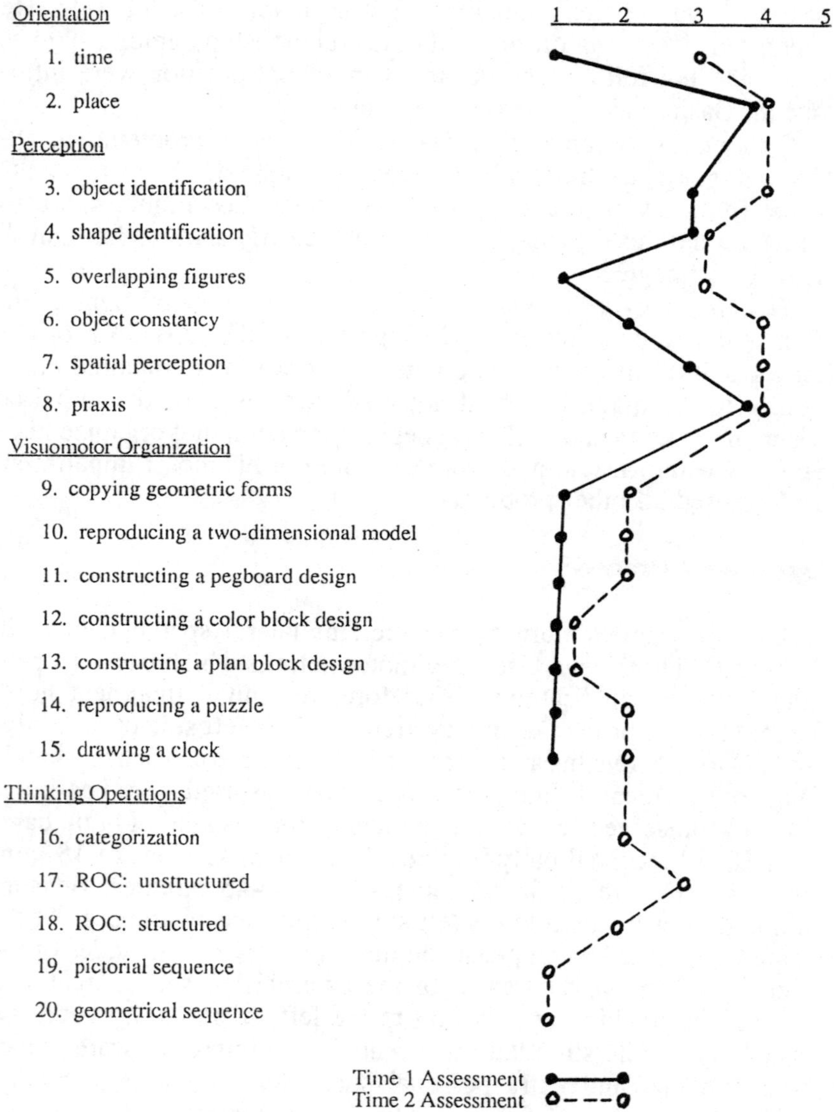

FIGURE 3. LOTCA Profile of CVA Patient for Two Assessments

First Assessment

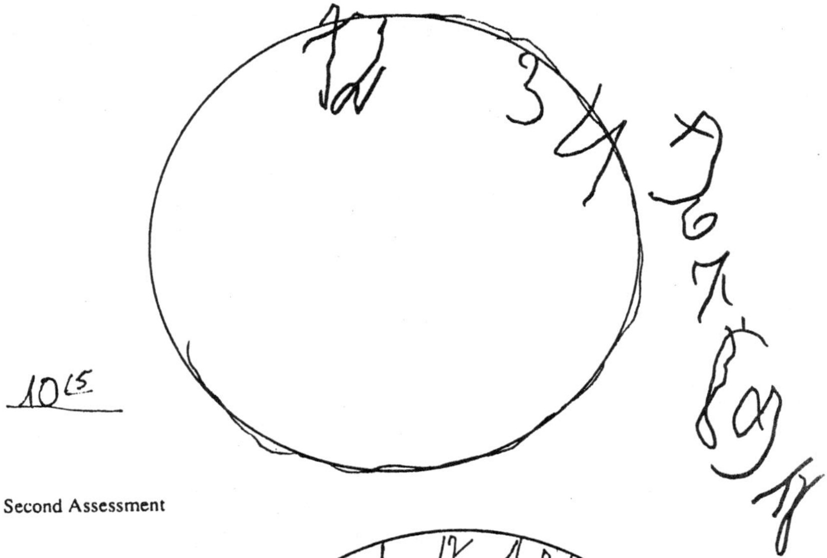

Second Assessment

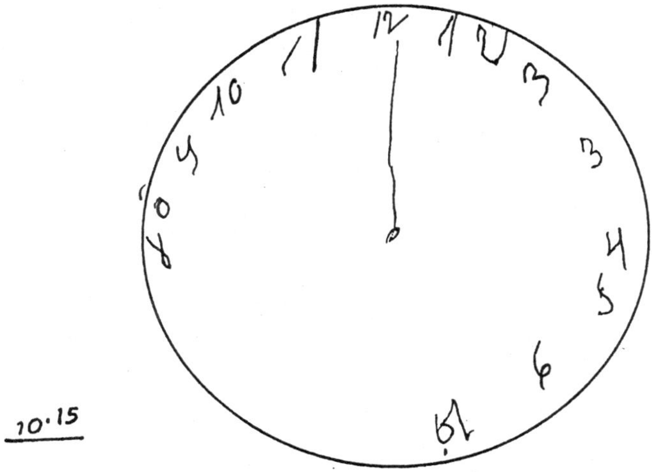

FIGURE 4. Examples of Clock Drawings of CVA Patient

ment to focus on more complex areas of visual perception and visuomotor organization. He still needed a lot of direction and cues. Additional goals included improvement of time orientation by working on a daily schedule and improvement of place orientation around the hospital.

Second Occupational Therapy Evaluation

A second evaluation was performed four months after administration of the first one. *Sensory motor* re-evaluation showed improvement in attending to auditory stimulus on the left. Equilibrium in sitting position was better, and David managed his wheelchair independently. He was also starting to walk with a four point cane and the support of another person. There was some movement in his left hand and a slight increase in tone. There was clear improvement in surface sensation but almost no improvement in proprioception, and tactile extinction existed when given tactile bilateral stimulation. The deficit in visual field remained only in the upper left quarter. *ADL* re-evaluation showed that David had regained bladder and bowel control, was independent in eating and was mobile via wheelchair in the hospital. He still needed some help in transfers and in bathing, and needed guidance and supervision in dressing.

Cognitive assessment: Summary of the LOTCA (see Figure 3) suggest improvement in almost all sub-tests. Most change occurred in visual perception with only slight improvement noted in visuomotor organization. At this time thinking operations could also be assessed due to increased attention span and concentration. However, performance in this area was comparably low to the visuomotor organization area. It appears that the deficit in both areas is dependent on impairment of perceiving and analyzing visual information.

In summary, there was improvement in all areas, but as a result of the location of the damage and especially the right subcortical damage, the rate of improvement was very slow and the expectations for full recovery are slim (Meshulam, 1985). At this time the rehabilitation plan was for David to return home under close supervision of his family. He will be able to walk at home but will need a wheelchair for longer distances. Further treatment will be given in the community with follow up at Loewenstein Hospital.

CONCLUSION

We presented two case studies, one of a young adult brain injured patient who suffered from a left lesion with aphasia and right hemiparesis, and the second an older stroke patient who suffered from a right hemisphere lesion causing a left hemiplegia with left unilateral spatial neglect. In the first case the visual system was better preserved and was capitalized on in the initial assessment and treatment, while in the second case the auditory input mode was utilized at first as it was the most preserved. Still, for both patients the same methods of evaluation were used, and the LOTCA provided a profile baseline for cognitive functioning and a measure of clinical change.

Both cases were described during the acute stage of their illness. Recovery at this stage is caused by spontaneous changes as well as by treatment effects, hence, no claim is made here to attribute the changes to the effectiveness of occupational therapy treatment methods alone. However, using an objective and detailed instrument to monitor progress proved to be extremely useful to the occupational therapy intervention process and to the therapists' reports within the interdisciplinary team. It should be noted of course, that an accurate assessment with the LOTCA cannot always be obtained due to patient's deficits in communication and/or attention, a limitation which seems to be inherent in almost all tests.

Still it is highly recommended that occupational therapists use measures for follow-up documenting clinical change in comparison to a baseline data in all areas, sensory motor, cognitive, and in daily activities. This supports Giles (1989) recent recommendation to use single subject experimental designs to demonstrate effectiveness of occupational therapy after severe brain trauma. Even though we did not adhere to a strict single subject design, and our purpose has not been to test occupational therapy effectiveness by itself, the use of ongoing assessments is essential and extremely important.

REFERENCES

Abreu, B.C. (1987). Rehabilitation of perceptual cognitive dysfunction. New York: A workshop manual.

Abreu, B.C, & Toglia, J.P. (1987). Cognitive rehabilitation: A model for occupational therapy. *American Journal of Occupational Therapy*, 41, (7), 439-453.

Almli, C.R. & Finger, S. (1988). Toward a definition of recovery of function. In S. Finger, T. E. LeVere, C.R. Almli, & D.G. Stein, *Brain injury and recovery*. New York: Plenum Press.

Averbuch, S. & Katz, N. (1988). Assessment of perceptual cognitive performance: Comparison of psychiatric and brain injured adult patients. *Occupational Therapy in Mental Health, 8*, (1), 57-71.

Averbuch, S. & Katz, N. (1989). Age level standards of the Loewenstein Occupational Therapy Cognitive Assessment (LOTCA). *American Journal of Occupational Therapy* (submitted).

Ben-Yishay, Y. & Diller, L. (1983). Cognitive remediation. In M.Rosenthal, E. Griffith, M.B.Bond, & J.D.Miller (Eds.) *Rehabilitation of the head injured adult*. Philadelphia: F.A. Davis.

Bernspang, B., Viitanen, M. & Reiksson, S. (1989). Impairment of perceptual and motor functions: Their influence on self-care activity 4 to 6 years after a stroke. *Occupational Therapy Journal of Research*, 9, (1), 27-37.

Carter, L.T., Howard, B.E. & O'Neil, W.A. (1983). Effectiveness of cognitive skill remediation in acute stroke patients. *American Journal of Occupational Therapy*, 37, (5), 320-326.

Carter, L.T., Oliveira, D.O., Duponte, J. & Lynch, S,V. (1988). The relationship of cognitive skills performance to activities of daily living in stroke patients. *American Journal of Occupational Therapy*, 42, (7), 449-455.

Fussey, I. & Giles, G.M. eds. (1988). *Rehabilitation of the severely brain-injured adult: A practical approach*. London: Croom Helm.

Giles, G.M. (1989). Demonstrating the effectiveness of occupational therapy after severe brain trauma. *American Journal of Occupational Therapy*, 43, (9), 613-615.

Giles, G.M. & Clark-Wilson, J. (1988). The use of behavioral techniques in functional skills training after severe brain injury. *American Journal of Occupational Therapy*, 42, (10), 658-665.

Golden, C.J. (1984). Rehabilitation and the Luria Nebraska neuropsychological battery. In B.A. Edelstein & E.T. Couture (Eds.) *Behavioral assessment and rehabilitation of the traumatically brain damaged*. New York: Plenum Press.

Inhelder, B. & Piaget, J. (1964). *The early growth of logic in the child*. New York: W.W. Morton.

Katz, N, Itzkovich, M, Averbuch, S. & Elazar, B. (1989). Loewenstein Occupational Therapy Cognitive Assessment (LOTCA) battery for brain injured patients: reliability and validity, *American Journal of Occupational Therapy*, 43, (3), 184-192.

Luria, A.R. (1973). *The working brain*. London: Penguin Books.

Meshulam, M. (1985). *Principles of behavioral neurology*. Philadelphia: F.A. Davis.

Najenson, T. Rahmani, L. Elazar, B. & Averbuch, S. (1984). An elementary cognitive assessment and treatment of the craniocerebrally injured patient. In B.A. Edelstein & E.T. Couture (Eds.) *Behavioral assessment and rehabilitation of the traumatically brain damaged*. New York: Plenum Press.

Neistadt, M.E. (1988). Occupational therapy for adults with perceptual deficits. *American Journal of Occupational Therapy*, 42, (7), 434-440.

Rahmani, L. (1982). The intellectual rehabilitation of brain-damaged patients. *Clinical Neuropsychology*, 4, (1), 44-45.

Siev, E., Freishtat, B. & Zoltan, B. (1986). *Perceptual and cognitive dysfunction in the adult stroke patient*. Thorofare NJ: Slack.

Soderback, I. (1988). The effectiveness of training intellectual functions in adults with acquired brain damage. *Scandinavian Journal of Rehabilitation Medicine*, *20*, 47-56.

Toglia, J.P. (1989). Visual perception of objects: an approach to assessment and intervention. *American Journal of Occupational Therapy*, 43, (9), 587-595.

Wechsler, D. (1981). *Wechsler Adult Intelligence Scale*. New York: Psychological corporation.

Ylvisaker, M. & Gobble, M.R. eds. (1987). *Community re-entry for head injured adults*. Boston: A College-Hill Publication, Little Brown.

Zoltan, B.B. & Ryckman Meeder, D. (1985). Head injury in adults. In L.W. Pedretti, *Occupational therapy practice skills for physical dysfunction*. St. Louis: C.V.Mosby.

Goal Attainment Scaling in Post-Acute Outpatient Brain Injury Rehabilitation

Barbara Zweber, OTR
James Malec, PhD

SUMMARY. Therapists continuously strive for efficiency in clinical practice. Goal Attainment Scaling (GAS) is a tool that can provide both a structure for objective documentation of patient progress and a means of program evaluation. This article describes the application of GAS in a comprehensive outpatient brain injury rehabilitation program. The benefits of GAS include: (1) objective data in monitoring participants' progress, (2) a structure for team conferences, (3) facilitation of ongoing rehabilitation planning and decision-making, (4) concise relevant information to funding sources, referral sources, and family members, and (5) a mechanism for program evaluation. For the brain injured person, GAS serves as a focus for an array of multiple, often abstract program goals. GAS can also increase the participant's awareness of deficits being addressed in the program and of progress towards resolving these problems.

INTRODUCTION

Occupational therapists strive to document therapeutic goals in measurable, graded sequences for the development of functional skills in daily living. In addition, therapists and/or program directors are increasingly aware of the need for a tool for program evaluation. Goal Attainment Scaling (GAS) is a tool that has been long used in mental health settings for program evaluation. Although

---

Barbara Zweber and James Malec are affiliated with the Mayo Clinic and Foundation.

GAS has not been as widely utilized to evaluate rehabilitation outcomes, its limited use in rehabilitation settings has generally received positive evaluations (see, for example, Clarke, 1983; Maloney et al., 1976; Sherman, 1985).

GAS is a method that simultaneously provides (1) a set of individualized goals and (2) outcome data that can be statistically summarized across all program participants. With minor modifications (for example, re-evaluating goal attainment every two weeks rather than only at program completion) GAS is being used in a comprehensive outpatients' program as an effective means of documentation and for program evaluation.

This paper will first describe GAS in general and then its application at the Mayo Outpatient Brain Injury Program emphasizing its use in documenting individual patient progress and as a program evaluation tool. A case history is included to further illustrate the use of GAS with brain injured people. What follows is a brief description of GAS. A more detailed review and discussion can be found in Smith (1981).

GOAL ATTAINMENT SCALING

GAS is a highly individualized system of outcome measurement that involves the use of a five-point scale. The expected outcome (long-term goal) is identified and becomes the zero point on the scale. Then other relative levels of goal attainment are placed on the scale in reference to this expected level of outcome. +1 and +2 refer to better than expected and much better than expected levels of outcome, respectively. −1 and −2 refer to levels of outcome that are, respectively, worse than and much worse than expected.

In order for the measurement procedure to be valid, levels of goal attainment must be stated objectively. Levels are objectively described in terms of concrete behaviors that can be observed and recorded. Table 1 provides two examples of writing goals using GAS. Between four and six discrete goals per individual are recommended.

Table 1: Examples of goal attainment scales

Orientation Group

Goal: Improve route finding ability

+2	Finds way among two or more community resources
+1	Finds way from hospital to two community resources
0	Finds way from hospital to one community resource
-1	Finds way from residence in hospital to therapy area and back
-2	Needs help to find therapy area from hospital residence

Social Awareness Group

Goal: To identify and accept my strengths and weaknesses, as indicated by thinking less about the way I used to be before my injury

+2	Thinks* about the way he used to be 2-3 times per week or less
+1	Thinks about the way he used to be about once per day
0	Thinks about the way he used to be 2-3 times per day
-1	Thinks about the way he used to be 2-3 times per hour
-2	Thinks about the way he used to be constantly, that is unable to be distracted from this thought

* as indicated by his spontaneous verbalizations

BENEFITS OF GOAL ATTAINMENT SCALING

There are a number of benefits in using the GAS in a brain injury program. One of the benefits is providing structure to the biweekly patient care conferences. At the care conference evaluation of goal attainment for each group, the brain injured person participates and is assessed for progress. Biweekly review of the individual's GAS provides a focus for the patient care conference and also provides a clear concrete indication of progress that is understandable to the program participants and families. In this way, GAS provides a mechanism that encourages insight into the patient's status and motivation for both patient and family. Another benefit of GAS is to illustrate the small increments in progress typically seen in brain injury rehabilitation.

Therapists working with brain injured persons utilize various outcome measure systems including the Glasgow Outcome Scale (Jennett et al., 1981), and the Ranchos Los Amigos Scale (Hagen, 1982). In the post-acute setting, the majority of patients show little or no progress on these scales because scaling is not sufficiently sensitive to reflect long recovery period and the complexity of functional deficits. In contrast, a therapist using GAS has greater potential to show the participant's progress because the measuring tool is personalized for each individual.

Goal scales are stated in measurable functional outcomes which constitute realistic levels of goal attainment specific to the individual patient. GAS also provides a structure for documentation, thus making it easier to provide objective data on progress to funding and referral sources. In addition, GAS makes it easy to track a patient's status (improve, decline, or plateau) and make appropriate plans and decisions regarding future rehabilitation efforts.

Another benefit of GAS is its applicability in program evaluation. Goal attainment only needs to be evaluated at program completion for purposes of program evaluation. In the ideal situation, an outside evaluator observes the program participant at program completion and rates the participant on his or her objective goal scales. Such a procedure of external evaluation provides the most objective method of program evaluation.

TREATMENT SETTING

The Mayo Outpatient Brain Injury Program is a rehabilitation program which emphasizes the development of social, cognitive, self-management, and vocational skills that are necessary to facilitate community re-entry. The outpatient program is similar to that described by Prigatano (1985). Participants attend the program five-days a week, spending the morning and early afternoon in the hospital-based interdisciplinary rehabilitation program and the late afternoon in individual therapy and/or community-based vocational activities.

The hospital-based rehabilitation program consists of six groups. Two occupational therapists facilitate the Orientation Group and the Cognitive Group, and one occupational therapist co-facilitates the

Communication Group with a speech pathologist. Other groups are the Self Awareness (psychotherapy) Group, the Leisure Skills Group, and the Fitness Group. The six groups are designed to promote cognitive skills and compensation techniques, self-awareness, social skills, emotional adjustment, pragmatic communication skills, leisure interests and skills, fitness, and health maintenance.

Employment or re-employment is the long term goal for most program participants, and is pursued through vocational evaluation, training, work simulation, and supported work trials. These vocational activities are provided by state vocational rehabilitation and local workshop services each afternoon after the hospital-based morning and early afternoon group sessions.

Families attend a biweekly group to facilitate their understanding and support of participants' activities in the program and their own emotional adjustment to the participant's disabilities.

APPLICATION OF GOAL ATTAINMENT SCALING

One long-term goal using GAS is developed for each group in which the brain injured individual participates. Because participant input, and hence, ownership of and commitment to the determined goals is highly desirable, goals are developed with as much input from individual participants as they are capable of providing. In the outpatient program, we arbitrarily set the initial level of goal attainment at which participants enter the program at -1. This allows for the possibility of regression to -2. The rehabilitation team does the scaling of each participant's goals on the five-point scale. Table 1 provides an example of goal attainment scales for the Orientation Group and the Social Awareness Group for one program participant who will be discussed in more detail in the Case Illustration section of this paper.

CASE ILLUSTRATION

The case history that follows further illustrates GAS with the brain injured population. Tom, a 39-year-old man with 3 children, suffered extensive brain injury in an automobile accident. Previous to entering the outpatient program Tom was involved in a comprehensive rehabilitation program for several months in a large midwest rehabilitation Center. Table 1 shows two examples of his six long term goals using the goal attainment scaling.

Figure 1, a stacked bar graph, illustrates Tom's progress in goal attainment in conjunction with other milestones of outpatient rehabilitation. Each vertical bar of the graph shows the combined levels of the six goal attainment scales for this individual for each month spent in the program. To reduce the size of the graph, GAS data are reported on a monthly basis, even though goal attainment was assessed every two weeks. The height of each of the variously marked sections of the vertical bars shows the absolute level (|1| or |2|) of goal attainment in each group. The position of the bar section above or below the zero line indicates whether the level is positive or negative. When the bar sections disappear from the graph, this indicates a zero level or expected level of goal attainment. The total bar shows overall goal attainment.

Figure 1 illustrates that progress, as indicated by GAS, was also reflected in progress in other outcome measures of outpatient reha-

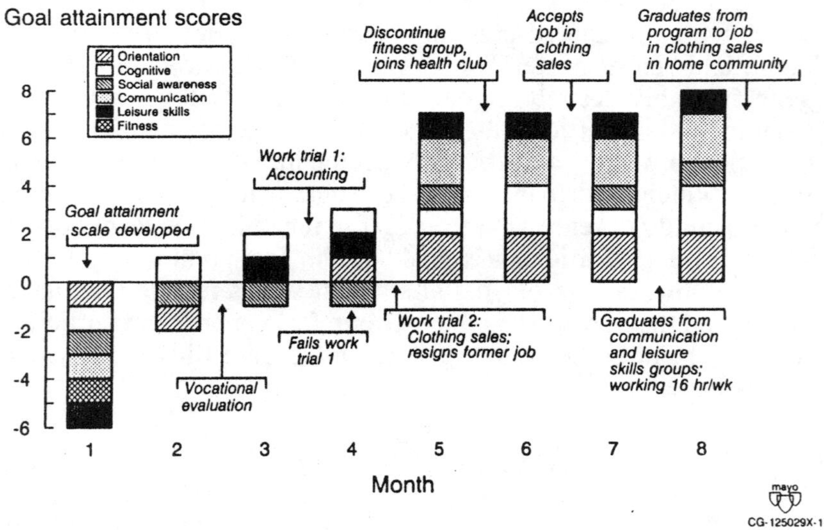

FIGURE 1. Goal Attainment Scaling and Other Milestones of Outpatient Rehabilitation

bilitation for this individual. The use of GAS facilitated making important decisions in Tom's rehabilitation planning. For example, as his route finding ability improved, as indicated by reaching an expected level of goal attainment in the Orientation Group (see Figure 1, month 3), the rehabilitation team felt comfortable involving him in vocational activities outside the hospital to which he travelled independently.

At another point in time (see Figure 1, month 5), Tom wished to discontinue the Fitness Group and join a health club. Again, the decision to allow him to do so was facilitated by GAS which indicated that he had reached an expected level of goal attainment in the Fitness group. Yet another example was when Tom had an opportunity to increase his hours at his part-time job (see Figure 1, month 7) and needed to decrease his involvement in the hospital-based program in order to do so. Because he had achieved a better than expected level of outcome in the Communication Group and a better than expected level of outcome in the Leisure Skills Group, the decision to graduate him from these groups and encourage him to use this time to increase hours spent at work was quite straightforward.

Tom had held an executive position prior to his brain injury. A major step for him in his outpatient program was to recognize that he was no longer able to perform his previous work because of his current cognitive disabilities. Tom's insight into his inability to return to his former job was increased through a work trial in which he attempted to perform some budgeting and accounting functions with supervision at the local sheltered workshop. Although his failure at this work trial was very distressing to him, working through his distress eventually resulted in progress (see Figure 1) on his goal in the Social Awareness group (i.e., "to identify and accept my strengths and weaknesses, as indicated by thinking less about the way I used to be before my injury"). In conjunction with his progress in the Social Awareness group, Tom was able to officially resign from his former position and accept a work trial placement in clothing sales at which he could be successful.

GAS also provides a method for facilitating participants' awareness of their progress. As Tom was working through his distress regarding his inability to return to his former employment, he became frustrated, feeling that he had gained little from the program. At this point, he was given the assignment of identifying his level of goal attainment on his personal goal scales. In general, his self-assessment of goal attainment was consistent with the assessment of the rehabilitation team. This self-assessment process using GAS helped him recognize his accomplishments in the program and regain the motivation to continue to pursue personal goals.

CONCLUSION

GAS is an effective method for monitoring and documenting participant progress and for program evaluation in post-acute brain injury rehabilitation. Using GAS, a highly individualized outcome measure can be developed which reflects goal achievement specific to each individual program participant. As important as individualized goal setting, the use of GAS in program evaluation allows for the computation of summary outcome date (e.g., mean, median, range, etc.) for groups of participants because all individualized goal scales use the same metric scaling system. GAS offers occupational therapists, along with other members of the rehabilitation team, a valid, quantified, and individualized assessment that provides (1) objective data in monitoring patient progress, (2) structure for team conferences, (3) assistance in rehabilitation planning and decision-making, (4) concise, relevant information for funding sources, referral sources, and family members, and (5) a method for program evaluation. In addition, the goal setting and monitoring process appears to increase staff's, patients' and families' understanding of outpatient program participants and how they change.

GAS provides the program participants with a concrete, individualized focus for multiple, more abstract program goals. As such, GAS facilitates the individual's insight into problems being addressed in the program. While participants accomplish a variety of smaller and short-term goals, GAS gives them feedback about their progress in the major milestones of their rehabilitation program.

REFERENCES

1. Clark, MS., Caudrey, DJ. (1983). Evaluation of rehabilitation services: the use of goal attainment scaling. *Internal Rehabilitation Medicine* 5, 41-45.

2. *Goal Attainment Scaling in Rehabilitation*. (1976) Chicago: Jewish Vocational Service.

3. Hagen, C. (1982) Disorganization following severe closed head injury; conceptualization In L.E. Trexler (Ed.), *Cognitive rehabilitation; conceptualization and intervention* (pp. 131-151). New York: Plenum Press.

4. Jennett, B., Snoek, J., Bond, M.R., Brooks, N. (1981). Disability after severe head injury, observation or the use of the Glascow Outcome Scale. *Journal of Neuropsychology, Neurosurgery and Psychiatry*, 44, 285-293.

5. Maloney, FP., Mirrett, P., Brooks, C., Johannes, K. (1978). Use of the goal attainment scale in the treatment and ongoing evaluation of neurologically handicapped children. *American Journal of Occupational Therapy*, 32, 505-510.

6. Prigatano, G. (1985). *Neuropsychological Rehabilitation after Brain Injury*. Baltimore: Johns Hopkins.

7. Sherman, R.G., Berling, B.S., Oppenheimer, S. (1985). Increasing community independence for adolescents with spina bifida. *Adolescence* 20, 1-13.

8. Smith, A. (1981) Goal attainment scaling: a method for evaluating the outcome of mental health treatment. In P. McReynold (Ed.), (pp. 424-59) *Advances in Psychological Assessment*. Vol 5. San Francisco: Jossey-Bass.

The TBIIM: An Intervention Model for the Treatment of Individuals with Traumatic Brain Injury

Elizabeth DePoy, PhD, MSW, OTR/L

SUMMARY. This article describes an intervention model for occupational therapists who treat individuals with traumatic brain injury. The model moves occupational therapy intervention beyond traditional skill acquisition in the clinical setting to the promotion of role function in the client's community environment. Concepts from the Model of Human Occupation, phenomenology and neurorehabilitation are integrated to provide the therapist with a set of guidelines for life-long intervention with individuals with traumatic brain injury. A case example is used to illustrate the model and implications for treatment and research are discussed.

With the increasing recognition of the life-long problems created by traumatic brain injury, rehabilitation professionals must now modify existing time-limited intervention models to promote greater functional capacity in this population. These models must include both formal rehabilitation and informal services after discharge. This article suggests an intervention model for individuals with traumatic brain injury (TBI). The Traumatic Brain Injury Intervention Model (TBIIM) is anchored on the integration of clinical observation with literature from neurology, rehabilitation and occupational therapy.

The article begins with a discussion of the assumptions and limitations of the model. The model is then described in detail, fol-

Elizabeth DePoy is Assistant Professor, Department of Social Work, University of Maine, 112 Annex C, Orono, ME 04469.

lowed by a brief case study to illustrate the application of the model to practice. The paper concludes with implications for practice and research.

ASSUMPTIONS AND LIMITATIONS

The model is limited to individuals with traumatic brain injury who have emerged from coma, are over the age of 16 and have moderate to severe impairment. These limitations have been imposed for several reasons. First, as supported by demographic data, the majority of head injuries occur in young adult males (Rosenthal et al., 1983). Secondly, the recovery process of individuals with mature nervous systems differs from that of children and thus, intervention models for children must consider a different recovery process than that of adults (Finger and Stein, 1982). As supported by contemporary research, the age at insult is a major determinant in the degree and nature of neurological recovery. Thirdly, the potential to attain a functional worker role, a goal most appropriate to adults, is a major focus of this model. While some of the tenets of the model can be applied to individuals with mild head injuries, this population has not been fully addressed by the TBIIM because these individuals do not frequently seek formal rehabilitation.

The model is based on three major assumptions: (1) early intervention; (2) the principle of meaningful intervention; and (3) the principle of life-long recovery, each of which is discussed below.

Early Intervention

As indicated by Finger and Stein (1988), Lezak (1979) and Prigatano (1986), who have proposed a holistic approach to rehabilitation strategies, the model assumes that rehabilitation be initiated as early as possible in the recovery process. While it was previously thought that the mature brain was static, contemporary research revealed that the dynamic nature of brain tissue renders the mature brain capable of regeneration after trauma (Bach-y Rita, 1988). Thus therapy may now be seen not only as compensatory, but restitutive.

Meaningful Intervention

The second major assumption is that relevant activity enhances patient participation in the intervention process. Thus, rehabilitation must take on a contemporary and expanded focus beyond the traditional hospital based approach. In essence, the rehabilitation team must move beyond the walls of the institution in both treatment planning and intervention if intervention is to promote life-long function. The rehabilitation team must also consider the unique life style and future living environment of each patient in planning relevant and meaningful intervention.

Life-Long Recovery

In order for rehabilitation to be meaningful in the lives of individuals with TBI, it must be a life-long effort. Individuals must be supported in their home, leisure and work environments throughout the lifespan. This time expansion therefore requires the rehabilitation team to develop new problem defining and resolving strategies. Rather than direct intervention following discharge from formal rehabilitation, the rehabilitation professional takes on the role of consultant to others who may provide support and structure in the client's living environments.

THE MODEL

The TBIIM is both a process and content model. It draws heavily on concepts from the Model of Human Occupation (Kielhofner and Burke, 1983). The foundation in human occupation is synthesized with principles of phenomenology and neurorehabilitation into a domain specific process of assessment, intervention goal setting, implementation, evaluation and modification for life-long intervention. Through using this model, the occupational therapist directs the intervention to the establishment of functional habits and routines upon which role function is based, while respecting the unique life style and experience of each individual.

Figure 1 depicts the content of occupational therapy assessment and treatment. Within this model, the occupational therapist must consider intervention from three distinct time perspectives; premor-

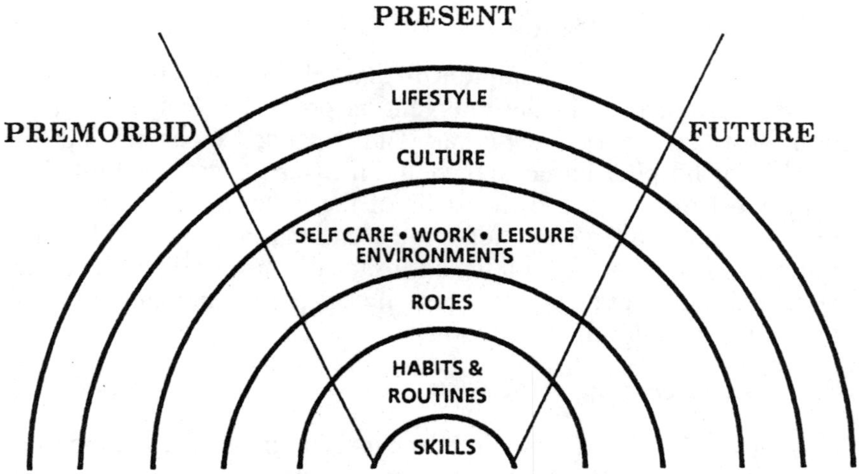

FIGURE 1. Content & Functional Level of OT Intervention

bid, current and future. In addition, six levels of influence on occupational function must be addressed.

Beginning with skills, the occupational therapist must consider current skills exhibited by the client in order to set goals for future skill acquisition. Once the skill level has been explored by the occupational therapist, the client's routines and habits require attention. The establishment of functional routines and habits which are consistent with individual life style is the major focus of the TBIIM.

Based on skill potential, the occupational therapist assists the client to modify and/or develop habits and routines that will prove functional in self care, leisure and work roles. For example, even if an individual is able, motorically and cognitively, to dress, dressing may not be functional in the home environment due to the common inability of individuals with TBI to generalize skills across environments. This model directs the occupational therapist to organize skills into functional routines in the environment in which the client will ultimately live. (See Figure 2 for depiction of the environmental levels accessed by clients.) Thus, each routine is expanded and practiced in each level of the environment that the client will encounter.

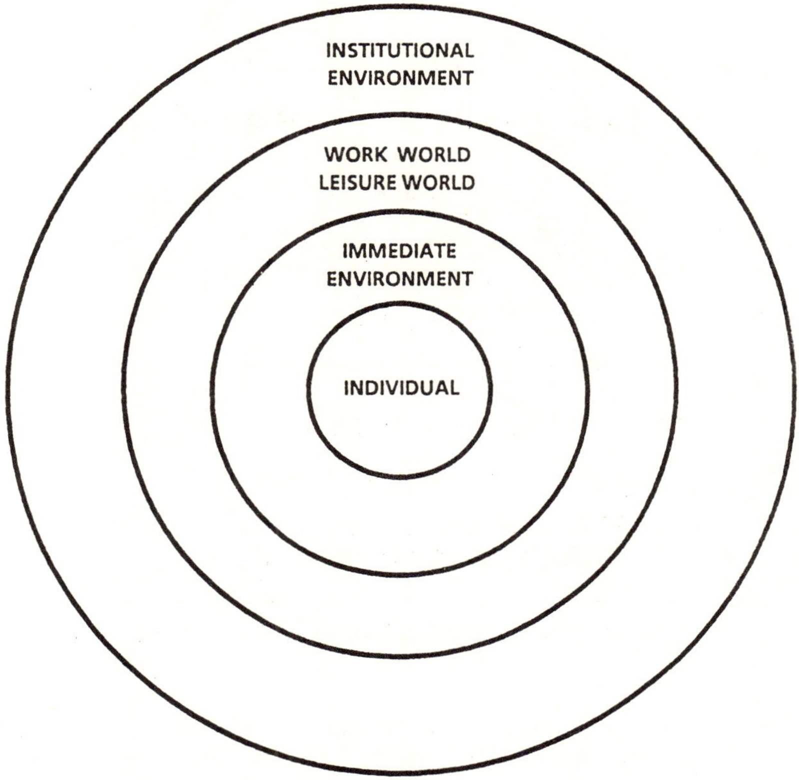

FIGURE 2. Levels of Person/Environment Interaction

The influence of culture and individual life style is also integrated into treatment, since the model assumes that clients are most likely to engage in familiar and personally relevant activity. In other words, the occupational therapist enhances the clients' ability to "do" activity in such a manner that the client is able to maintain uniqueness while regaining a balance of work, leisure and self care roles in all levels of his/her living environment.

Figure 3 depicts the process of occupational therapy intervention. The aim of intervention is the acquisition of functional roles which serve the client in varied environments while preserving individual style. The role of the occupational therapist is to apply his/her pro-

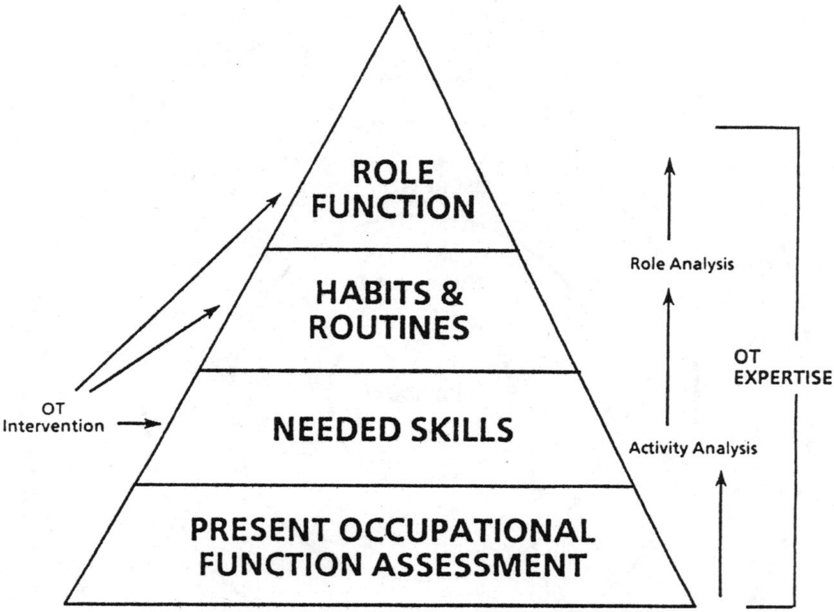

FIGURE 3. Sequence of Facilitating Role Acquisition

his/her professional expertise to promote role acquisition through hierarchical steps of skill development and subsequent organization of skills into functional routines required to perform life roles.

The first step of the process is assessment. Assessment must consider premorbid occupational status and predicted future status. The assessment procedures should be structured to answer the question "What do I need to know about this patient's past, present and future in order to plan and implement the most effective intervention?" While most occupational therapists are familiar with the skill or performance level of assessment, an occupational therapist, as part of the rehabilitation team, does not have to administer all skill assessments. Information on past, present and potential skill return can be obtained from other team members. For example, the neuropsychologist can give a much more detailed and comprehensive picture of cognitive function than the occupational therapist, since cognition is a fundamental domain of neuropsychology. The social worker is most likely to possess the premorbid information, including psychosocial function, family history and living environments. The focus of occupational therapy assessment should be in the area of expertise that the occupational therapist possesses, namely that of occupational function. Therefore, the most critical levels of occupational therapy assessment are in the area of routines and role function. While not widely available, some standardized assessments of role function, habits and routines do exist. For example, the KELS (Kohlman Evaluation of Living Skills (McGourty, 1979) and the Role Checklist (Oakley, 1981) are two assessments developed by occupational therapists that examine occupational role function and have undergone validity and reliability study. However, interview and observation in task behavior is essential to supplement and amplify quantitative assessment information.

In addition to assessing occupational performance, the OT assesses the patient's need for environmental structure and modification. Due to the nature of traumatic brain injury, skills easily executed in a controlled clinical setting may not be easily accomplished in other settings. For the patient who is assessed as independent in dressing in the clinical setting but unable to dress in his/her room, valuable and necessary intervention is omitted if the occupational therapist fails to rehearse routines and make necessary modifications in the non-clinical environments in which the patient performs. The nature of occupational therapy assessment provides an excellent mechanism for evaluating what a patient "does" as opposed to what a patient should be capable of doing. In the TBIIM the occupational therapist uses activity and task performance as the basis for assessment in which patients are required to demonstrate function within an appropriate and normative environmental setting.

A brief example of work assessment illustrates the value of task performance. The occupational therapist may create a simulated work environment in which work etiquette, often a major area of difficulty for an adult with frontal lobe injury, can be evaluated. By asking an individual to function as part of a work team, the ability to work with others, follow directions, and exhibit a functional work style can be observed.

Task performance in a simulated setting may reveal deficits

which would prevent an individual with intact cognitive and motor skill from functioning competently in a work environment. That is to say, task performance should be used to evaluate areas of work performance which cannot be ascertained on standardized work skill assessment. Without task performance, an individual who might be recommended for competitive employment may be at risk for failure if deficits in areas such as temporal orientation, social judgement and self-monitoring are not identified and remediated. The ability to conduct a valid and reliable assessment through simulated activity is dependent on the occupational therapist's systematic approach to data collection and analysis.

Once an assessment has been completed, the next step of the occupational therapy process, goal setting, begins. Based on the six levels of influence on role function depicted in Figure 1, the occupational therapist structures goals and operationalizes them into objectives which guide intervention and specify outcome criteria. Goals suggest a structure for the timely acquisition and organization of skills and routines into functional roles. For example, a goal might look something like; Client will practice and refine mathematical computation and money handling as a basis for the self care role of grocery shopping. In the TBIIM, each goal statement must specify the role that it addresses and the environment in which the role is to be enacted. In this manner, intervention moves beyond the skill focus.

The right-hand side of Figure 3 depicts occupational therapy processes and areas of expertise which are used in translating goals into intervention. Once again, the focus of the TBIIM is on the promotion of habits and routines which will promote normative role acquisition and adaptation to multiple environments. The TBIIM expands the basic occupational therapy skill of activity analysis into role analysis. In activity analysis the therapist reduces activity into its smallest parts, while in role analysis, the parts of a role are identified and integrated with the environmental elements which guide role function. Thus, the desired roles, revealed in the comprehensive assessment, are translated into organization of skill and routines within specified environments.

Intervention begins with the acquisition of new skills, which is accomplished by designing a program of incremental skill mastery.

However, skill acquisition by itself falls short of the focus of the TBIIM. The model guides the occupational therapist to provide intervention which enables the client to organize mastered skills into varied and functional routines in the client's living environment. Further, the intervention activities must be relevant to client life style and needs.

As the intervention is implemented, the occupational therapist assesses outcome, both formally and informally. Formal measures may involve evaluating the degree of change from initial assessment to current time on standardized instruments and task performance.

In addition, the occupational therapist continually seeks information about the extent to which the intervention is enhancing the client's capacity to exercise roles relevant to his/her unique lifestyle. This information may sometimes only be ascertained by observing role function in actual living environments. For this reason, the rehabilitation team must begin to expand intervention and assessment beyond the institution. As the client reintegrates into the community, continued outcome assessment will redefine treatment modifications. The primary aim of life-long intervention is to decrease professional services to the minimal level of support necessary for clients to resume productive lives. While professional involvement may be extended over a longer period of time, the ultimate results of life-long support are to reduce crises requiring reinstitutionalization and to promote productivity.

To summarize, the assessment process in occupational therapy focuses on the two fundamental elements of role function: the status of habits and routines, and the environments in which roles will be enacted. While skill assessment may be necessary, it is likely that much information may be obtained from other team members and need not be repeated by the occupational therapist. The living environments of clients are identified and assessed for structure necessary for the client with TBI to perform functional role behavior.

The TBIIM guides intervention which is aimed at the acquisition of context specific role function which recaptures the unique life style of each client. Following the termination of formal rehabilitation, the occupational therapist should remain involved in intervention as long as needed to promote the continuation of person-environment fit in the client's desired roles.

CASE EXAMPLE

Using the model, the following case describes intervention for a moderately head injured 30-year-old male patient with predominantly left hemisphere sequelae. He was admitted as an inpatient in a rehabilitation hospital setting six weeks following emergence from a coma. Formal assessment included administration of the Weschler Adult Intelligence Scale by the neuropsychologist, the Weschler Memory Scale by the occupational therapist, a family history taken by the social worker and observation of task performance in simulated work, self care and leisure situations in the occupational therapy clinic. Assessment of skill revealed that the client demonstrated intact fine and gross motor skills but exhibited mild adynamia (an executive cognitive function which prevents the initiation of action), social disinhibition, poor social judgement and inability to perform problem solving at the formal operational level. Information processing was slow, impairing new learning, and long term semantic and episodic memory was mildly impaired. At the routine level, the client exhibited disorganized behavior insufficient to allow function in self care, work or leisure unless he was directed to every task in a highly structured environment.

After having obtained formal assessment data, the occupational therapist learned, through interview, that the patient wanted to return to his premorbid job of computer operator. With these impairments, however, it was unrealistic to set such a goal before improving role function in less complicated environments and without considering the need for supervised or supported employment in the distant future. The goals set for this patient therefore considered skills, routines and habits necessary for life-long function in the third environmental level of work and leisure. (See Figure 3.)

Based on initial assessment data, the client's first set of inpatient goals were :

1. patient will explore memory devices and strategies as a basis for development of routines to compensate for memory and initiation deficits which interfere with role development at all environmental levels;
2. patient's living environment will be adapted to provide external memory and temporal cues which promote initiation of self care roles;
3. patient will routinize the use of external memory and temporal cues as a basis for following a daily schedule, promoting role function in the leisure and work levels of the environment;
4. patient will develop a morning self care routine to include bathing, dressing, and arriving at the dining area on time as a basis for establishing a normative worker schedule and role in the work level of the environment;
5. patient will engage in supervised leisure activity with two or more persons in order to receive feedback on strengths and weaknesses in social judgement and in preparation for work and friendship role function in work and leisure environments; and
6. patient will participate in a variety of computer tasks in his immediate environment to explore his present level of computer skill and potential to develop functional computer routines for future remunerative roles in the work level of the environment.

These initial goals specified the environments in which the client would explore, enact and master skills necessary for role function in his future. The activities included computer retraining, recreational social games consistent with the client's life style and dressing and hygiene routine acquisition. The ultimate direction of intervention with this patient was the internalization of routines such that he would be able to initiate a balance of roles within supportive, structured living environments.

Evaluation of outcome for this client was ongoing through his inpatient rehabilitation stay. Upon discharge, the occupational therapist made a home visit with the social worker and goals were revised to address the client's role function in his home and in a simulated work program at the rehabilitation setting. Currently, the client is able to enact self care routines sufficient for independently arriving at his simulated job site on time for three days each week. On alternate days, the client spends mornings at a local health spa, where he is able to function at the leisure environmental level with minimal supervision. Future intervention will involve the client in socialization roles in his immediate and leisure environments and will aim towards supported employment in the distant future. The projected level of life-long treatment by an occupational therapist is consultation to lay persons and work supervisors to insure appropriate environmental structure. Yearly assessment of role function may continue until the client has returned to a balance of role functions in the environments in which the client's life style is enacted.

IMPLICATIONS

The TBIIM suggests guidelines for contemporary occupational therapy practice. Using the model, the occupational therapist moves from an outdated model of treatment to a contemporary community oriented focus. This change in intervention is appropriate both to the needs of brain injured adults and to the financial constraints of the health care system.

The use of such a model insures that the occupational therapist addresses the client's actual rather than potential performance. Because individuals with TBI often experience inability to transfer routines across environments, this model guides the therapist to rehearse and routinize behavior in all environments in which the client will interact. In addition, the need to provide intervention which is relevant to life style increases the likelihood of client investment in the treatment process.

From the financial perspective, the model directs the occupational therapist to implement intervention which is accountable and the aim of which is to return clients to maximum productivity. The role of consultant in life-long intervention reduces the cost of occupational therapy intervention while still providing necessary services.

The TBIIM is based on the belief that the foundation of occupational therapy lies in its unique focus on occupational function. Evaluation research should be conducted to refine the model and to modify it to more effectively meet the intervention needs of individuals with traumatic brain injury. However, research to develop occupational therapy theory should also be accomplished using intervention based on this model as a domain of inquiry.

REFERENCES

Bach-y-Rita, P. (1988). *Traumatic brain injury*. New York, Demos.

Finger, S. and Stein, D.G. (1982). *Brain damage and recovery: Research and clinical perspectives*. New York, Academic Press.

Kielhofner, G. and Burke, J.P. (1983). *Health through occupation*. Philadelphia, F.A Davis.

Lezak, M. (1979). Recovery of memory and learning functions following traumatic brain injury. *Cortex, 15*: 63-72

McGourty, L.K. (1979). Kohlman evaluation of living skills. *Intermim Manual*. Seattle, University of Seattle.

Oakley, F.M. (1981). *The role checklist*. College Park Maryland, Oakley.

Prigatano, G. (1986). Higher cerebral deficits: The history of methods of assessment and approaches to rehabilitation, Part II. *BNI Quaterly, 2*(3):15-26.

Rosenthal, M., Griffith, E.R., Bond, M.B., Miller, J.D. (Eds) (1982). *Rehabilitation of the head injured adult*. Philadelphia, F.A Davis.

Family Intervention with the Traumatically Brain Injured Patient

Jane Painter, MHS, OTR/L

SUMMARY. The occupational therapist plays an integral role in the evaluation and treatment of the traumatically brain injured (TBI) patient. Although the TBI patient's needs are relatively well-defined by the nature of the injury, less well recognized and frequently overlooked is the emotional and psychological trauma experienced by the family of the TBI patient. Depending on the information provided, the family can be an asset or hindrance in the patient's rehabilitation. By working with the TBI patient's family, the occupational therapist can guide the family into a more cohesive force that will assist the patient throughout the rehabilitative process. This article provides suggestions to evaluate and manage concerns and fears raised by the families of TBI patients. It provides an organizational guideline for educating the family about TBI and incorporating them in the rehabilitation of the TBI patient.

INTRODUCTION

The impact on families of individuals who have sustained a traumatic brain injury (TBI) has been well documented (Frye, 1982; Mathis, 1984; Mauss-Clum, 1981; Cope and Hall, 1982). Reac-

---

Jane Painter is Assistant Professor, Department of Occupational Therapy, School of Allied Health Sciences, East Carolina University, Greenville, NC 27858-4353.

The author wishes to express thanks to Dr. Robert Lust for his editorial assistance in reviewing the manuscript. The traumatically brain injured patients and families at West Florida Regional Medical Center, Pensacola, FL and Lutheran Hospital, Fort Wayne, IN, were instrumental in providing the clinical insight necessary to develop this review and the materials it contains.

tions include severe anxiety, denial, anger, withdrawal from other family members, poor decision making skills, rigidity, low frustration tolerance, and guilt (Johnson and Higgins, 1987; Rogers and Kreutzer, 1984; Zegeer, 1981). The significance of the crisis is in part a result of the role the TBI individual has in the family unit and the dynamics among the family members.

Factors that have influenced the family's ability to handle the crisis situation are dependent on the severity of injury, previous experience with illness, coping skills, family dynamics, and the quality of education provided at the early stages of hospitalization (Johnson and Higgins, 1987; Oddy, Humphrey, and Uttley, 1978; Orto, 1984; Mathis, 1984; Rogers and Kreutzer, 1984). Although the needs of families of TBI people have been studied (see for example Mauss-Clum, 1981; Mathis, 1984), little has been written about the family's involvement in treatment

The purpose of this paper is to briefly review the occupational therapy role in TBI family intervention and to present a family intervention program structured on the eight cognitive functional stages of recovery identified in the Rancho Los Amigos model (Trombly, 1989).

STAGES OF FAMILY RESPONSE TO THE TBI

To better understand how to facilitate family involvement in treatment, the stages of response to TBI need to be considered. The author has found that each family member of the TBI individual will progress through various stages that lead to the acceptance of the injury that are similar to the acceptance stages of death and dying (Kubler-Ross, 1969). Family members may not proceed at the same pace or through the suggested sequence of acceptance of their relative's TBI. For example, an individual family member's acceptance level may reverse as the relative's progress fluctuates.

Because brain injuries are typically caused by a traumatic accident, the family has had no forewarning and is initially in a state of shock and denial. Immediately after the accident, the family members may feel overwhelmed, helpless and numb, and function as though they are in an isolated tunnel.

Communication with family members may be difficult during

this stage. Information may need to be repeated and/or adapted before they understand what roles the various health professionals (e.g., physicians, nurses, and therapists) will play in the patient's recovery as well as in their own lives. The duration of this stage will vary for the individual family members and will depend on individual coping skills and the family support system as well as information provided by the medical team. The TBI individual's precarious prognosis also affects progression to the later stages (Rogers and Kreutzer, 1984).

The second stage involves feelings of anger, guilt, and depression. The family members may be angry at the TBI individual for the turmoil the members are experiencing but at the same time feel guilty for being angry. During this stage, the family members may focus their anger on the medical staff and each other rather than direct their anger at the TBI person. Depression usually follows anger and guilt. At this time, the family members may feel overwhelmed, frustrated, exhausted, and demonstrate decreased coping skills.

The third and final stage is acceptance of the traumatic brain injury. This implies that family members have a realistic understanding and acceptance of the TBI's physical, psychological, and sociological deficits, assets, and future prognosis. As the TBI person's health fluctuates so too will the family members' acceptance level. The family may also have unresolved feelings of isolation associated with the first stage of shock and denial. It is important to remember that each stage is not discrete and that feelings from previous stages may carry-over to the next stage.

ROLE OF THE OCCUPATIONAL THERAPIST

A major role of the occupational therapist (OTR) throughout the rehabilitation process is educating family members about the recovery process and their role in teaching and reinforcing desired behaviors (Rao, Sulton, Young, & Harvey, 1986). This starts in the Intensive Care Unit (ICU) when the OTR begins the evaluation and treatment process. The family's lack of education about the injury, what is being done to the patient, and what they as individuals can do intensifies their fears of the unknown and hinders their coping skills, often placing them on an "emotional roller coaster." However, the OTR can assist the family regain equilibrium by skill building through a comprehensive educational program (Frye, 1982). Idealistically, all team members should utilize the same approach in meeting the needs of both the TBI patient and family.

The first area of family intervention involves factual education of family members. This may include basic anatomical information about what has happened as a result of the TBI; the information about treatment modalities should be presented in lay terms. Information provided must reflect the acceptance stage(s) of the family member(s) as well as the most appropriate learning style for each individual. The factual education may include visual materials (pictures in books, brain models, slide presentations), written material (e.g., handouts or pamphlets) and/or audio suggestions (e.g., cassette tapes or music).

The second area of family intervention is the therapist's role as a model for interacting with the TBI patient. Role modeling of the staff occurs in this phase of learning which assists the family members to diminish their fears of the haunting equipment and noises found in the patient's room. By observing the OTR and other disciplines touch the patient and move the tubes and intravenous lines, family members learn that they cannot hurt their relative by touching the person or the attached medical paraphernalia. Therefore, the fear produced by strange equipment and noises in the patient's room is lessened, and the family is much more comfortable around their TBI relative.

The third important area of family intervention is to teach the family members various treatment procedures that they can perform while visiting. The OTR should consider the family members' educational level as well as acceptance stage before involving them in this area. To reduce the amount of stress and energy expended by the family member, the OTR should only provide one or two ideas per day. A complete outline of materials and suggestions for family involvement, organized according to the cognitive level of the TBI patient, is presented in the next section.

Needs differ for the children and adult relatives of the TBI person. Recent research has focused primarily on the needs of the adult family members of the TBI person (Mathis, 1984; Molter, 1979;

Mauss-Clum, 1981). Children often are neglected and/or confused about what is happening since they are not allowed to visit the ICU. Activities that would incorporate siblings in the TBI patient's occupational therapy program may include making or gathering items for the patient's hospital room or taping their voices talking or singing. Educating the children and involving them in the family support groups (if appropriate) is also a very beneficial way to help them cope with their fears.

FAMILY INTERVENTION PROGRAM FOR THE TRAUMATICALLY BRAIN INJURED PATIENT

The following family education section is based on the author's ten years experience with TBI patients and a literature review. This educational supplement incorporates the Occupational Therapy Performance Model (Punwar, 1988) and is structured according to the Rancho Los Amigos Adult Cognitive Functioning Scale (Trombly, 1989). It is designed as a handout to family members but is useful as a treatment guide for therapists as well. The suggestions in each cognitive functioning level are directed towards family member involvement.

This family instructional program should be used in a sequential order starting with the present functional level of the TBI patient. Keep in mind that each family member may be at a different acceptance level of the patient's injury and require a different approach to learning the individualized treatment plan. It is *impossible* for the entire program to be carried out during one visit. The term *you and your* used throughout refers to the family members.

LEVEL I (no response): At this stage, the patient appears to be in a deep sleep. Although the patient may be restless, he or she is unresponsive to all stimuli including pain, noise, or visual images.

LEVEL II (generalized response): At this level, the patient inconsistently responds to repeated sounds by becoming more or less active. The patient may also pull away from any pain causing stimulus, such as tracheotomy, IVs, catheter, and/or feeding tube.

FAMILY SUGGESTIONS FOR STIMULATION FOR LEVELS I AND II

1. Particularly in the beginning stages of recovery from a TBI, the patient may respond more to family members and close friends than to hospital staff. For this reason, it is important for family and friends to involve themselves in stimulating and orienting the patient as his or her tolerance permits. Remember, both the family and TBI patient require the proper amount of rest.
2. Part of the treatment plan consists of *sensory stimulation*. This should be performed at frequent intervals for 5-to-10 minutes throughout the day. Attempt to provide only one stimulus at a time, and try to appeal to various senses throughout the day. With each type of stimulation, describe what you are doing before, during, and after the activity. There may be a delayed response to the stimulus provided and it may be affected by your voice, body scent (e.g., body perfume or soap), jewelry, and color of clothes you are wearing. Here are some suggestions you can do during visiting hours:

   a. *TOUCH SYSTEM*: This is also called the tactile system and is one of the first systems to develop.

      1. Use firm rather than light pressure when touching the patient.
      2. Rub various textures on the arms, legs, and stomach using a firm pressure. Agitation may occur if the the face is touched with the various textures (cotton, silk, tissue).
      3. Assist the patient in touching his or her face, legs, arms, and/or stomach with his or her hand. Self-stimulation feels different compared to being touched by someone else.
      4. Bath time is an excellent opportunity to provide touch stimulation by using the wash cloth, towel, soap, and shampoo.
      5. Remember to talk to the patient and describe your intentions before the actual movement/touch.

b. *OLFACTORY SYSTEM*: This system refers to the sense of *smell* and plays an important role in providing sensory stimulation. The sense of smell has a close connection with your emotions. For example, the smell of freshly cut grass or certain foods may bring on pleasant memories while other smells may bring on bad memories. Here are some suggestions for the olfactory (smell) system:

1. This system may not be aroused if the patient has a NG (nose) feeding tube.
2. Use scented hand lotion when giving touch stimulation using a firm pressure.
3. When you visit, wear the patient's favorite cologne, perfume, or after shave lotion.

c. *VISUAL SYSTEM*: This system refers to *eyesight*. Please inform the medical staff if the patient wears glasses, contacts, and/or has visual problems.

1. You may stimulate the visual system (eyes) by bringing in family photographs (with names identified on the back so the staff will know who they are), posters, or mobiles.
2. Carefully select items placed by the patient's bedside. Please check with the nursing staff before you bring in too many items.

d. *AUDITORY SYSTEM*: The auditory system refers to *hearing*. Please inform the medical staff if the patient wears a hearing aide and/or has a hearing problem.

1. Cassette recordings of family members and friends may be used by the the staff throughout the day and evening.
2. Tell the specified multi-disciplinary treatment member the type of TV shows, radio station, and music the patient enjoys and dislikes.
3. When providing sensory stimulation or doing exercises tell the patient your intentions about *hearing* you do the actual movement.
4. Do not leave the radio or TV on longer than 10-to-15

minutes at a time since the patient can eventually tune out the sound.

5. Pay attention to your voice so you are not talking "baby talk." No one knows for sure how much someone in Levels I and II can hear so try to be positive and *not* talk about problems at home or how the patient looks.
6. Talking loudly will not help the patient hear better, but speaking in a variety of tones may increase the level of alertness.
7. Talk slowly by prolonging the pauses between your words and phrases.
8. Verbal communication can be improved by using effective gestures, facial expressions, and other visual cues.
9. Do not expect responses to questions, rather provide information to the patient.

3. *EXERCISE PROGRAM*: A special exercise program you can do during your visiting hours with the patient will be developed by the occupational and physical therapists. You will be given written and verbal instructions and demonstrations until you feel comfortable performing the exercises.
4. Continue to show affection in whatever manner you feel comfortable. The nursing staff, therapists, or other hospital personnel will instruct you about the various machines and/or tubes that are attached to the patient.

LEVEL III (Localized response): At this level, the patient is usually out of ICU and will begin to react specifically, but inconsistently, to stimulation. The response is directly related to the type of stimulation presented, as in turning the head toward a sound or focusing on an object. The patient may sporadically follow simple commands in a delayed manner such as closing the eyes, squeezing a hand, or opening the mouth. The patient may also show vague body awareness by responding to discomfort by pulling at the nasogastric tube, tracheotomy, catheter or resisting restraints. There may be a tendency to respond more to family members and friends.

At Level III, the patient will probably begin a more active therapy program to one or two times in the rehabilitation department. Time spent in therapy will depend on the patient's endurance and will last approximately 15-to-30 minutes for each discipline. As the patient's endurance improves, the therapy time will increase. If desired, a family tour of the rehabilitation department may be arranged.

FAMILY SUGGESTIONS FOR ACTIVITIES FOR LEVEL III

1. During this stage, purposeful response to commands and objects is emphasized. Noisy and confusing backgrounds may distract the patient from concentrating on the activity.
2. The radio and/or TV should be turned on for short intervals of 10-to-15 minutes to maximize the patient's attention span.
3. It is helpful to have the room as controlled as possible and eliminate visual distractions. Pulling the curtain around the bed may be of help, but check with the nursing staff first as the nurse may need to observe the patient.
4. Talk to the patient at eye level and within the patient's field of vision. Sit if necessary and assume a relaxed posture as this will convey your patience and willingness to "listen."
5. Limit the number of visitors to one or two people at a time. Encourage visitors to come in the evening hours when the patient is not participating in nursing or therapy activities.
6. Ask the patient to follow one-step commands, such as "open your mouth," "close your eyes," "show me your teeth," "raise your arm," "shake your head," "tap your foot," "rub your nose," "touch your hair," "give me your hand," "move your finger," "stick out your tongue," and/or "give me a big smile."
7. As the patient becomes more alert, ask questions that have "yes" or "no" answers. Allow ample time for the patient to respond.
8. Provide assistance to the patient in performing routine, self-care activities. These activities may include combing/brushing hair, washing face, and putting on lotion. A mirror may assist the patient in successfully executing the activity.
9. If *permission* has been received from the patient's therapists

or nurses, assist the patient with drinking from a cup or eating finger foods.

10. Orienting the patient to time, person, and place should be done throughout the day and evening. You can offer orientation information specifically and matter-of-factly. Each time you see the patient, introduce yourself, talk about what month, day and year it is, and where and why the patient is in the hospital. It is helpful to use family pictures, places, or objects to orient the patient.
11. When a patient has had a TBI, memory is usually affected to some degree. Past memory is the first type of memory to return after a TBI. Therefore, orientation of familiar things is essential. For example, talk about family members and long-time friends, personal address, type of work, hobbies, and/or interests. Do not expect the patient to answer specific questions, and making demands will not help the healing brain function better.

LEVEL IV (confused-agitated): A heightened state of activity with no behavioral awareness or control are the primary characteristics of this fourth level of TBI. The patient does not discriminate between persons or objects and is unable to directly cooperate with therapy efforts. The patient lacks short-term memory, and if able to speak, his or her communication may be inappropriate or not understandable. The patient requires moderate-to-maximal encouragement to perform self-care activities. This seems to be the most difficult stage for staff and families to cope with since the patient is unlike his or her former self. Often patients are antisocial. It is important to remember that the patient is not consciously trying to be obnoxious. This transitional stage is a sign of improvement and may be thought of as step toward recovery. Family members should request specific suggestions for coping with the patient's inappropriate behavior from the multi-disciplinary team.

FAMILY SUGGESTIONS FOR ACTIVITIES FOR LEVEL IV

1. The main goal at this level of confusion/agitation is to help channel the patient's excessive energy, attempting to tire the

patient during the day so it is easier for him or her to sleep at night. Walking with the patient (with the help of one or two other people) is an excellent way for the patient to expend extra energy. Please ask the physical therapist for *permission* to walk with the patient. If unable to walk, push the patient in a wheelchair while describing your location. This may have a calming effect. Be sure that the nursing staff knows where you are taking the patient and how long you will be gone.

2. The staff will gradually be increasing the patient's sitting tolerance. Your encouragement and conversations while the patient is sitting up may decrease his or her stress. The patient may forget how long he or she has been sitting up due to poor memory.
3. Ask for *permission* prior to removing any restraints on the patient since they are for the patient's own protection. If removed, caution must be taken so that the various tubes are not pulled out by the patient. Be sure to replace the restraints with verbal reassurance to the patient before you leave the hospital room.
4. Use the non-agitated moments for improving the patient's ability to appropriately respond to your questions and/or commands. Attempt activities in which the patient can succeed such as pointing to body parts, colors, objects in the room, family members or play catch with a nerf ball.
5. Encourage the patient to attempt simple self-care tasks such as brushing the teeth, washing the face, combing/brushing the hair, or putting on hand lotion. You may need to begin the activity and then ask the patient to complete it. Provide gentle and sincere praise for what the patient can perform. Give one activity at a time with simple commands and allow plenty of time for completion of the activity. The occupational therapist can help you with these activities.
6. Assistance at mealtime may be provided by properly positioning the patient, preparing the food so the patient can eat with help, and adjusting the room so there are few distractions. The dietitian will work with the patient and family to determine his or her food preferences. Check with the nursing staff to determine if the patient's liquid intake and output are being measured. The occupational and/or speech therapist can offer sug-

gestions if the patient has difficulty chewing, swallowing, and/or sucking.
7. Orientation to person, place, and time should continue and inappropriate responses should be corrected.
8. Having the patient wear a watch will assist in orientation. A watch indicating the date and displaying a bold, easy to read face and second hand is helpful.

LEVEL V (confused-inappropriate) The patient appears alert and is fairly consistent in responding to simple commands. Attention span is minimal and the patient will need frequent re-direction back to the task. The patient may be able to do automatic activities such as eating and dressing, but display difficulty learning new information. Agitation may appear when there is too much environmental stimulation.

FAMILY SUGGESTIONS FOR ACTIVITIES FOR LEVEL V

1. Continue to orient the patient to person, place, and time. Talk to the patient's therapists for memory enhancement suggestions.
2. Review biographical and family information with the patient. Discuss with him or her current problems resulting from the TBI honestly, accurately and matter-of-factly. This information will need to be repeated many times due to the patient's poor short-term memory.
3. Encourage the patient to find his or her room when walking or pushing self in the wheelchair about the hospital's floor.
4. Encourage the patient to succeed at each task, emphasizing what was accomplished and providing praise for each successful step of the activity. Be observant of the patient's attention span and frustration and fatigue level so that the activity does not become too overwhelming.
5. Keep candy and other "fattening" foods to a minimum. Frequently, the TBI patient will overeat or eat the wrong kind of foods and gain unwanted pounds. Fresh fruits are a good substitute for candy.

6. The patient's therapists may ask you to help your relative with assigned "homework" in the evenings and weekends.

LEVEL VI (confused/appropriate): The TBI patient is now capable of following simple directions consistently, and with supervision, is able to perform routine daily living skills such as eating, dressing, and bathing. Memory for recent events is still poor which interferes with new learning. However, past memory continues to improve. The patient no longer wanders in the hospital's hallways and is inconsistently oriented to time, person, and place. The patient may recognize some staff members and have an increased awareness of self, family, and basic needs. Attention span has increased to approximately 30 minutes.

FAMILY SUGGESTIONS FOR ACTIVITIES FOR LEVEL VI

1. The patient's independence may be increased by gradually decreasing the amount of assistance provided.
2. Continue using various activities such as crafts, games, sports activities with increasing complexity to help the patient with short-term memory and self-esteem.
3. As with Level V, assist the patient with "homework" that has been assigned by the therapist(s).
4. Ask the patient how to get from home to very familiar places such as work, school, friends' home, mall, or the grocery store.
5. Ask the patient what steps are necessary to perform various activities. This may be done in the hospital or at home when the patient has a weekend pass. (e.g., making a bed, setting the table, or using the dishwasher)
6. Limit the patient's TV time. Ask the patient to summarize what he or she just saw on the television.
7. Other activities that may help the patient prepare for discharge include money concepts, making change, using a vending machine, ordering food in the cafeteria, finding names and/or companies in the phone book, or ordering an item from a catalog.
8. Everyday activities that are taken for granted may be difficult

and frustrating for the TBI patient. It is important to use routine situations within the patient's tolerance level as a learning experience. You can assist the patient in problem-solving through each phase of daily living activities.

LEVEL VII (automatic/appropriate): The patient in this stage appears appropriate and oriented within the hospital and at home. Daily routines are performed automatically with minimal or no confusion. There is an increased awareness of self, body, family, foods, and the environment. However, the patient may lack insight into the TBI, display decreased judgment, problem-solving abilities, and unrealistic planning for the future.

Learning new information will occur but at a much slower rate. The patient will most likely will require supervision for safety purposes, for example when using the stove. Usually, the patient will be independent in self-care activities and with assistance be able to initiate social or recreational activities. Judgment remains impaired and the patient may be unable to drive a car or ride a motorcycle. Prevocational and avocational evaluations and counseling may occur at this stage.

FAMILY SUGGESTIONS FOR ACTIVITIES FOR LEVEL VII

1. Discuss with the patient situations within the home that could be potentially dangerous and the actions needed in case of an emergency.
2. Have the patient practice using the phone book, phone, and how to dial the police or emergency number(s).
3. Assist the patient in making a grocery list and finding the items at the grocery. Also, have the patient handle the money at the check-out lane.
4. A driving evaluation may be appropriate (with physician's order) if the patient continually insists he or she is able to drive. The rehabilitation department may be able to assist you with this task. If the patient is found to be eligible to drive, notify the Department of Motor Vehicles that your relative has had a TBI and will need to retake both the written and driving tests. It is also advisable for you to notify your insurance company to

see if there are any restrictions relevant to your family member.

5. While at home, have the patient perform daily routines such as make the bed, work in the yard, clean the house, or do the dishes.
6. To help the patient's short-term memory, judgment, and problem-solving skills, continue to use crafts, cards, games, and/or sport activities.
7. To increase the patient's ability to cope with stress and frustration, allow ample time to answer questions and/or problem-solve.

LEVEL VIII (purposeful/appropriate): At the final stage, the patient is alert, oriented and can recall and integrate recent events. Poor memory of the early phase of the TBI may occur. The patient is most likely able to drive and is independent in home and community skills. An evaluation by vocational rehabilitation will determine the patient's abilities to return to work. The patient may continue to show decreased ability to reason, tolerate stress or noise, and/or use good judgment in emergency or unusual situations.

FAMILY SUGGESTIONS FOR ACTIVITIES FOR LEVEL VIII

1. Encourage maximum involvement in the home and the community within the patient's physical/emotional abilities.
2. If unable to drive, the patient will need assistance with public transportation until independence is attained.
3. A referral should be made to the Department of Rehabilitation Services (DORS) if the vocational rehabilitation counselor determines that the patient cannot return to work. This agency provides counseling services, pre-vocational testing, and funds for continuing education or buying special/adapted equipment.
4. If needed, encourage the patient to become responsible for independently taking the prescribed amount of medication.
5. Encourage the patient to prepare his or her own budget, appropriately use charge cards, write checks, and balance the checking account as financial responsibility improves.

6. Continue increasing the difficulty of leisure and daily living activities to help improve the patient's frustration tolerance, short-term memory, and problem-solving skills.

CONCLUSION

The OTR has an important role in identifying and alleviating the TBI family's fears, anxieties, frustrations, and acceptance of their relative's condition. Through a comprehensive educational program with the OTR, the family members become active participants in the TBI's treatment. This includes factual education, role modeling, and facilitating family involvement in treatment. Information provided by the OTR should be based on the individual family members' acceptance and educational levels as well as the needs of the TBI patient. This paper has presented a family education program to teach family members about TBI and to facilitate their involvement in the treatment process.

REFERENCES

Cope, D. & Hall, K. (1982). Head injury rehabilitation: benefit of early intervention. *Archives Physical Medicine Rehabilitation, 63*, 433-437.

Dunkel, J. & Eisendrath, S. (1983). Families in the intensive care unit: their effect on staff. *Heart and Lung, 12*(3), 258-261.

Elliot, J. & Smith, D. (1985). Meeting family needs following severe head-injury: a multidisciplinary approach. *Journal of Neurosurgical Nursing, 17*(2), 111-113.

Frye, B.(1982). Brain injury and family education needs. *Rehabilitation Nursing, Jul-Aug*, 27-29.

Johnson, J. & Higgins, L. (1987). Integration of family dynamics into the rehabilitation of the brain-injured patient. *Rehabilitation Nursing, 12*(6), 320-322.

Kubler-Ross, E. (1969). *On Death and Dying.* NY, NY: MacMillan Publishing Company.

Livingston, M., Brooks, D., & Bond, M. (1985). Three months after severe head injury: psychiatric and social impact on relatives. *Journal of Neurology, Neurosurgery, and Psychiatry, 48*, 870-875.

Mathis, M. (1984). Personal needs of family members of critically ill patients with and without acute brain injury. *Journal of Neurological Nursing, 16*(1), 36-44.

Mauss-Clum, N. & Ryan, M. (1981). Brain injury and the family. *Journal Neurosurgical Nursing, 13*(4), 165-169.

Molter, N. (1979). Needs of relatives of critically ill patients: a descriptive study. *Heart and Lung, 8*(2), 332-339.
Oddy, M., Humphrey, M., & Uttley, D. (1978). Stresses upon the relatives of head-injured patients. *British Journal of Psychiatry, 133*, 507-513.
Orto, A. (1984). Coping with the enormity of illness and disability. *Rehabilitation Literature, 45* (1-2), 22-23.
Punwar, C. (1988). *Occupational practice: Principles and practice.* Baltimore, MD: Williams and Wilkins.
Rao, N., Sulton, L., Young, B., & Harvey, R. (1984). Rehabilitation team and family assessment of the initial home pass. *Archives Physical Medicine Rehabilitation, 67*, 759-761.
Rogers, P. & Kreutzer, J. (1984). Family crises following head injury: a network intervention strategy. *Journal of Neurosurgical Nursing, 16*(6), 343-346.
Sherburne, E. (1986). A rehabilitation protocol for the neuroscience intensive care unit. *Journal of Neuroscience Nursing, 18*(3), 140-145.
Trombly, C. (1989). *Occupational therapy for physical dysfunction*, 3rd edition (p. 487). Baltimore, MD: Williams and Wilkins.
Zegeer, L. (1981). The patient in the persistent vegetative state. *Journal of Neurosurgical Nursing, 13*(5), 243-247.

A Descriptive Study of Family Directed Therapy for Traumatically Brain Injured Persons

Laura Harvey Krefting, PhD, OT(C)

SUMMARY. Long term outcome after traumatic brain injury is a major concern for rehabilitation professionals, family members, and the general community because of the complex residual physical, social, cognitive and psychological problems associated with the disability. This paper reports the findings of an exploratory study investigating the nature of caregiving provided by family members in the community. Family directed therapy (FDT) is defined, and data about 22 informants' patterns of FDT activities are described. The similarity of FDT to occupational therapy practice is discussed and implications for facilitating caregiver involvement in FDT described.

Traumatic brain injury has been termed a "silent epidemic" in health care and is rapidly becoming one of the most active areas of specialization in rehabilitation (Namerow, 1987; Rosenthal, 1984). Recent medical and technological advances have created a group of long term survivors who exhibit severe physical, social, emotional and cognitive limitations. Moreover, these numbers are escalating because of rapid social change as evident in drinking and driving patterns and risk-related leisure activities. Importantly, because of the complex and enduring nature of the residual problems, the majority of brain injured people are unable to function independently and many return to their natal families. Family caregivers, most

---

Laura Harvey Krefting is Associate Professor, School of Rehabilitation Therapy, Queen's University, Kingston, Ontario K7L 3N, Canada.

The author is indebted to the informants for giving of themselves and to Susan Zikiwsky and Linda Miller for their contributions to this study.

often aging parents, are then responsible for the long term care of the disabled individual.

The significance of family caregiving practices was one of the results of an ethnographic study conducted to determine the long term outcome of traumatically brain injured individuals (Krefting, 1989). The majority of family caregivers interviewed in the study provided some type of therapy for their disabled family members at home, even those injured 20 years previously. These activities included exercise programs, problem solving tasks, and games to promote cognitive skills. These home-based activities by caregivers are termed family directed therapy (FDT). Family directed refers to the fact that responsibility for developing, maintaining and evaluating therapy belongs to the family rather than professionals. Moreover, little if any professional input is sought or offered.

The purpose of the study described here was to explore and further define the concept of FDT identified in the ethnographic research. First, background literature on the family and brain injury will be summarized. A brief description of the study will be followed by the presentation of the results and a discussion of the implication of the study to occupational therapy practice.

RATIONALE AND REVIEW OF LITERATURE

Family directed therapy is important because professional services are discontinued, typically after the first two years after the injury, and any gains made after that are predominantly through the efforts of the family caregiver. As Kovich (1985) notes, the length of time spent in a medical facility may be minimal compared to the time the patient will spend recovering in the home. Family caregiving is also important because as Livingston, Brooks, and Bond (1985) state, in many cases new problems appear in the years following the injury long after rehabilitation services have stopped. For example, reactive psychiatric problems may develop in response to the long term nature of the disability. Families, then, are forced to use their own resources to address these new problems in addition to the residual limitations.

The majority of literature on families and brain injury focuses on the family as recipient of therapy rather than on their role as providers of therapy after discharge. A number of studies have documented the effects of the brain injury on the disabled person's family members (Hopewell, 1985; Oddy, Humphrey and Uttley, 1978; Thomsen, 1984), which include depression, anger, and often family break-up. The importance of intervention with the family was described over a decade ago by Lezak (1978) in a seminal paper on living with the brain injured patient.

An example of literature which focuses on the family as "patient" is Diehl's (1984) chapter on family education. Describing the importance of the patient and family as equal partners in the rehabilitation process, she cites a number of interventions for the family including reality orientation, family conferences, and educational groups. She does not, however, address the idea of teaching educational approaches to family members as an intervention itself.

In the same volume, Rosenthal and Muir (1984) note the importance of family intervention. They illustrate the impact of the disability on the family and describe three categories of professionally initiated techniques for addressing family problems: patient-family education about brain injury, family counselling, and family therapy. Rosenthal and Young (1988) later build on the idea of family intervention by describing four additional types of intervention: marital and sexual counselling, family support groups, family networking, and family advocacy. Klonoff and Prigatano (1987) also note the reactions of the family members to traumatic brain injury and describe family involvement in the rehabilitation process as one means of addressing maladaptive reactions. They describe involvement with professionals as a way of orienting family members to the nature of professional rehabilitation and providing them with a more realistic idea of the brain injured person's abilities. Although they support family participation in therapy at the rehabilitation center, involvement is viewed primarily as beneficial for the family (as an intervention) rather than as a way of transferring therapeutic skills to the family.

DePompei, Zarski, and Hall (1988) present an approach to involve families in cognitive-communication rehabilitation that is intended to be carried on at home. Based on family systems theory, they describe a model of dysfunctional family reactions to the injury and outline interventions to minimize these reactions. They suggest professionals have pre-discharge practice sessions with family which include rehearsal and role playing (with video) of techniques for cognitive communication problems such as reframing and constructive feedback. Although their approach helps prepare family caregivers for living with the brain injured person at home, they also stress that family members must retain their roles as family members and not be given the role of a professional and the responsibility for therapeutic intervention.

McKinlay and Hickox (1988) present an approach that recognizes the family as a resource in treatment in describing the family member as a co-therapist after discharge from hospital. Their study focused on techniques meant to reduce memory failure and temper outbursts in the brain injured person using family members as co-therapists. Rather than simply providing counselling and education, they identified the need for family to be actively involved in treatment in both the early stages of recovery and later in the transitional stage. Although they describe one means of involving family in therapy, they do not address the critical issue of family member as the only therapist after discharge from rehabilitation.

Kovich (1988) comes the closest to addressing the idea of FDT in her description of home programs as part of the discharge process. She outlines a number of principles that facilitate following home programs prescribed by the rehabilitation team prior to discharge. She suggests providing family members with treatment goals, methods of grading activity, and photographs of exercises or proper wearing of adaptive equipment.

In summary, the literature on families of brain injured people focuses largely on family reactions to brain injury and methods of treating the family. The small number of references to family participation in therapy come from an institutional context where the family caregiver is a member of the rehabilitation team, most often in the earlier stages of recovery. There is little information available about the nature of therapy that is conducted by family caregivers in the absence of professional supervision.

METHOD

This descriptive study used structured interview methodology to explore the nature of FDT. First, a comprehensive literature review was undertaken to identify material on family caregiving for traumatically brain injured people as well as other disability groups.

Relevant data from a previous study on long term outcome after traumatic brain injury was reviewed. Based on the literature, the ethnographic data, and clinical experience, a structured interview schedule was developed. The schedule was reviewed by two individuals experienced in interview methodology, pilot tested on three family caregivers not included in the sample and then revised before use in the study.

The subject pool, one of convenience, was the membership of the local head injury foundation. Members were contacted by an individual not involved in the research project by telephone and asked if they would be willing to be interviewed about caregiving in the home. Interviews were conducted in the informants' home when the disabled family member was not present. The same researcher conducted all interviews. Interviews averaged 1 1/2 to 2 hours in length.

Responses to the specific items on the interview schedule were written during the interview and general impression and data extraneous to the schedule but relevant to FDT were noted. Interview data was transferred onto computer and the responses categorized and frequencies derived.

RESULTS

Informants

Twenty-two caregivers were interviewed which included: 8 parents, 12 spouses, and 2 siblings of brain injured individuals. Nineteen informants were female and 3 were male. The average age of caregiver was 45 years. The length of time that informants had been caregivers ranged from under 1 year to 24 years; 8 had been caregivers under 1 year, 7 between 2 and 5 years, 3 between 6 and 9 years, and 4 had been caregivers for over 10 years.

In addition to demographic information about the caregiver and family member, descriptive information was gathered about the functional level of the brain injured person which included: activities of daily living (ADL), communication, energy level, and behavior. Although no standardized outcome instrument was used, brain injured individuals can be roughly classified as mildly impaired (10), moderately impaired (7) and severely impaired (5).

None of the brain injured persons were employed. All caregivers reported their family members had "problem" behaviors which ranged from uncontrollable outbursts and antisocial behavior to social isolation.

Nature of FDT

Nineteen of the 22 caregivers interviewed were involved in FDT. The three informants not involved in FDT cited the brain injured person's lack of motivation as the reason. However, in all three cases, the family caregiver had attempted some type of therapy at home but had abandoned the activity when there was no response.

The types of FDT activities provided by the caregivers fell into six major areas: therapeutic ADL (15), recreation (13), socialization (12), specific cognitive activities (10), physical exercises and therapy (10), and therapeutic games (6). Examples of activities included: carpentry projects, helping with "work book" exercises, practicing telephone use, setting up social situations and providing feedback, and making weekly job lists. The majority of informants were involved in at least two different types of activity. A typical pattern of FDT activities included: supervised exercise routine and feedback on social and communication skills on a daily basis and weekly recreational activity. Sixteen informants described scheduling of daily and weekly activities as an important part of FDT.

Almost all caregivers attempted to make therapeutic situations out of ordinary activities. For example, one informant described swimming on Saturday morning as:

> It is more than just an outing. It is therapy because we do certain special exercises and then we discuss how he did with the exercises and also the social stuff. But we would do it anyway even if he wasn't hurt.

Another example of making therapeutic opportunities out of common experiences is using ADL as "therapy." As one informant noted:

> Doing the vacuuming or making a sandwich—trying to do it the right way, the most efficient way without distraction. Just the thought process she has to come up with to get the result. Practice like that makes great therapy.

Consistent with the emphasis on FDT reflecting ordinary activities, special equipment was reported used in FDT by only four informants. One purchased adapted eating equipment and three informants obtained special "school" materials which contained cognitive retraining types of exercises.

Although most FDT activities were conducted on an ad hoc basis, 7 caregivers planned specific "therapy time," similar to the pattern followed in a rehabilitation center. For example most caregivers involved in physical exercises scheduled two 30 minute periods, one in the morning and one in the afternoon.

Informants had difficulty specifying how much time they spent in FDT activities because many of the activities were incorporated in routine patterns. For example, one informant gave feedback on behavior several times a day and helped with exercises. When asked to make a rough estimate of time spent, 3 informants stated they were involved in FDT 1-3 hours weekly and the remaining 16 informants provided FDT on a daily basis; 8 informants provided it 1-3 hours daily, 2 informants provided it 4-6 hours daily, and 6 informants provided over six hours daily.

Thirteen of the 22 caregivers reported that other family members participated in FDT activities although the informant was the initiator of activities. One caregiver had assistance from a part-time housekeeper and two informants described family friends as being involved in helping carry out FDT activities.

One interview item explored where caregivers learned how to do FDT activities. Ten of the 19 informants reported that the FDT activities were their own invention. Several commented that there had been no formal discharge program to instruct families how to care for the disabled person at home. The other nine informants based FDT programs on advice given by health care professionals: 7 from occupational and physical therapists, 1 from a physician, and 1 from a teacher.

Another interview item referred to the family member's level of motivation to participate in FDT. Seventeen of the 19 caregivers providing FDT and the 3 informants that were not involved in FDT found that motivating the brain injured person was a problem.

To gather data about caregiver perceptions of FDT effectiveness, informants were asked about the criteria used to determine if FDT worked. Responses included: increased independence (7), more appropriate behavior (7), improved social skills (5), increased level of activity (3), and increased initiation of activity (3). Informants were asked whether the family member had improved since discharge from rehabilitation. Thirteen informants felt that progress had been made, and 10 informants attributed the improvement in part to FDT. Interestingly those caregivers who thought no progress had been made continued their FDT activities despite their having no apparent effect.

DISCUSSION

FDT appears to be a reaction both to the family's sense of responsibility for doing all that is possible for the disabled person and also to the inadequacy of existing community services for brain injured individuals. As one informant noted when the family member was discharged from the rehabilitation center: "OK, now what do I do? You realize there is no one. It is all up to you."

As reported in the general literature on caregiver burden, almost all caregivers are women; in this case most of them were older mothers of brain injured young men. To be responsible for an adult son functioning much like a child is a difficult task. Several caregivers reported that their lives had reverted to a pattern similar to that of having small children at home, a stage in life they thought far behind them.

The nature of FDT seems associated with the disabled person's stage of recovery. The more recently the disabled person had been discharged from hospital the more likely it was that caregivers reinforced therapy exercises seen at hospital or "homework" given when the disabled person was an outpatient. The 10 informants who reported FDT was based on professional advice had been caregiving under five years. As regular contact with professionals stopped, FDT seemed to take a new form that required greater effort and creativity. All of the informants who reported that they had no discharge help and had devised the FDT on their own had been caregivers for over five years. The comparative lack of rehabilitation services at that time or the caregiver's inability to remember that period are possible reasons for this.

One interesting aspect of the interview data was the importance of what I term the "cultural appropriateness" of FDT activities. The majority of caregivers' injured family members were young men, and caregivers strived to develop activities which were appropriate for their sons or husbands, things that the disabled person might have done had he not been injured.

> Trying to get him back to society—the only thing I could think of that was appropriate for an old lady (mother) and a young guy was to go to restaurants. So we ate our way through those first years at home.

Another caregiver developed a therapy program for her son at a health spa. She mixed exercises she had seen in the rehabilitation center, those she had seen on television and exercises others at the spa were doing, into her own "therapy" program. She felt that at least going to the spa was normal activity for a 25-year-old man even if he was in a wheelchair.

The similarity of the FDT described here and occupational therapy activities is obvious. The use of therapeutic ADL activities reflects the functional emphasis of occupational therapy which is one of the basic tenets of the profession. The emphasis of FDT on "ordinary activities" also reflects occupational therapy principles. For example the frequency of FDT recreational types of activities suggest that caregivers are seeking a way of structuring the day (the concept of temporal adaptation) and of providing a legitimate role. Although this preliminary study did not focus specifically on the rationale behind the choice of FDT activities, several informants spontaneously described the problem of the family member "having nothing to do and no where to go." Many informants reported that the majority of injured family members' time was spent in front of the television. The recreational activities were also seen as one way of replacing employment. The use of recreational activities as a substitute for competitive employment suggests that caregivers are using the concept of meaningful occupation as seen in the following interview excerpt.

> I racked my brain to come up with something for him to do that was useful—that would occupy my husband's time—something besides TV all day long. Then I struck on collecting bottles.

This caregivers innovative "job" for her husband, collecting bottles and soda cans four hours daily and keeping records of amount of money earned, exemplifies many of the basic tenets of occupational therapy and emphasizes the complex nature of family directed therapy.

PRACTICE IMPLICATIONS

Although the preceding discussion draws attention to the similarity between FDT and occupational therapy, I am not advocating that family caregiving can replace occupational therapy in long term treatment after traumatic brain injury. Rather, the therapist has a critical role in enhancing the caregiver's ability to provide FDT on a long term basis.

One strategy is to teach basic therapeutic principles to families before the disabled individual is discharged from therapy; for example, the principles of grading an activity, basic activity analysis, appropriate ways to provide feedback and support, and methods of monitoring progress. This education program can be extended by developing a series of video tapes that caregivers could borrow or purchase to reinforce what is taught by the therapist.

A preventive approach with caregivers is another way that therapists can enhance FDT. Recognizing the heavy burden placed on caregivers, it is important to prepare the caregiver for the "burn out" frequently created by long term caregiving (McKinley & Hickox, 1988). Family members need to have a realistic picture of the demands on the caregiver months and years after their family member is discharged from rehabilitation. The therapist can assist the caregiver in establishing a social support system and in identifying the types of support that will be necessary for long term caregiving. Therapists can also alert caregivers to the signs of burnout and suggest community resources for use when needed. In addition, health promotion activities and respite strategies should be addressed.

In preparation for teaching caregivers about FDT, occupational therapists need to assess the family's ability to be therapeutically supportive and to direct ongoing therapy. Included in this assessment is the caregiver's ability to interact with the patient, his or her learning style, and comprehension of the understanding of the likely prognosis of the disability.

In the ideal health care system, regular long term follow-up provides the therapist with the opportunity to meet with the brain injured person and the family caregiver in the home environment. With such extended contact, the therapist could assess the effectiveness of FDT and offer suggestions and new techniques when necessary. This is rarely financially feasible, however, so occupational therapists must optimize their opportunities to work with family caregivers while the injured family member are in active treatment.

LIMITATIONS OF STUDY

This study was a preliminary, explorative study into the nature of FDT and as such has some limitations. The applicability of the findings to the larger population of caregivers is limited because of the small sample size. In addition, the sample was one of convenience and is not necessarily representative because it was drawn from a family support organization. Caregivers belonging to such groups are more likely to be involved with the family member than caregivers who are not members of a support group. The fact that 19 out of 22 informants were involved in the same type of FDT can not be interpreted as incidence and should not be generalized beyond this descriptive study.

CONCLUSIONS

Although the families of traumatic brain injured persons have been described in terms of their reactions to injury and intervention to address family problems, little information exists about family caregivers as providers of therapy. This study is a first step in describing the nature of long term family directed therapy for survivors of traumatic brain injury. The findings suggest that families develop a repertoire of ways to manage the experience of brain injury and to promote recovery. Many of these FDT activities make use of the principles underlying occupational therapy. The family is key to the long term outcome of traumatically brain injured people. As such, enhancing their therapeutic abilities should be one of the goals of occupational therapy with traumatically brain injured persons.

REFERENCES

Diehl, L. (1984). Patient-family education. In M. Rosenthal, E. Griffith, M. Bond, & J. Miller (Eds), *Rehabilitation of the head injured adult* (pp 395-406). Philadelphia: F. A. Davis Company

DePompei, R., Zarski, J., & Hall, D. (1988). Cognitive communication impairments: A family-focused viewpoint. *Journal of Head Trauma Rehabilitation*, *3*, 13-22.

Hopewell, C. A. et al. (1985). Long term family disintegration after head injury. A comprehensive treatment approach. *Journal of Clinical and Experimental Neuropsychology*, *7*, 1948-1949.

Klonoff, P. & Prigatano, G., (1987). Reactions of family members and clinical intervention after traumatic brain injury. In M. Ylvisaker, & E. Gobble (Eds) *Community re-entry for head injured adults*, (pp 381-402) Boston: Little, Brown and Company.

Krefting, L. (1989). Reintegration into the community after head injury: The results of an ethnographic study. *Occupational Therapy Journal of Research*, *9*, 67-83.

Kovich, K. (1988). Family education and discharge planning. In K.Kovich, & D. Bermann (Eds.) *Head injury: A guide to functional outcomes in occupational therapy*, (pp. 205-210). Rockville: Aspen Publishers.

Lezak, M.D. (1978). Living with the characterologically altered brain injured patient. *Journal of Clinical Psychiatry*, 592-598.

Livingston M. G., Brooks, D. N. & Bond, M. (1985). Patient outcome in the year following severe head injury and relatives psychological and social function. *Journal of Neurology, Neurosurgery, and Psychiatry*, *48*, 876-881.

McKinlay, W. & Hickox, A. (1988). How can families help in the rehabilitation of head injured? *Journal of Head Trauma Rehabilitation*, *3*, 64-72.

Namerow, N. S. (1987). Current concepts and advances in brain injury rehabilitation. *Journal of Neurologic Rehabilitation*, *1*, 101-114.

Rosenthal, M. & Muir, C. (1984). Methods of family intervention, In M. Rosenthal, E. Griffith, M. Bond, & J. Miller (Eds), *rehabilitation of the head injured adult* (pp 395-406). Philadelphia: F. A. Davis Company.

Rosenthal, M. & Young, T. (1988). Effective family intervention after traumatic brain injury: Theory and practice. *Journal of Head Trauma Rehabilitation*, *3*, 42-50.

Executive Function and Cognitive Remediation: A Study of Activity Preference

Elizabeth DePoy, PhD, MSW, OTR/L
Kathleen Maley, OTR/L
Joanne Stanraugh, OTR/L

SUMMARY. Through the use of multiple case study design, this project examined the variations in executive function exhibited by two subjects who sustained frontal lobe damage. The study then investigated the relationship between executive functional deficit and activity preference. Subjects were trained in computerized cognitive retraining and conventional cognitive retraining. Subjects were then asked to select either modality. Each subject was tested for initiation and overall executive function, cognitive status and disability level. Findings revealed that executive functional deficits present in varied and unique ways and that activity preferrence is related to the unique constellation of sequelae rather than location of injury. Further implications point to the value of combining informal and formal inquiry techniques to patient assessment as well as research on closed head injury intervention.

As the incidence of closed head injury increases, efforts to remediate chronic disability resulting from closed head injury (CHI)

Elizabeth DePoy is Assistant Professor, Department of Social Work, University of Maine, 122 Annex C, Orono, ME 04469. At the time this study was conducted, she was a member of the faculty of Occupational Therapy Department, Thomas Jefferson University, Philadelphia, PA. Kathleen Maley was Occupational Therapist on the Brain Injury Rehabilitation Unit, Magee Rehabilitation Hospital, Philadelphia, PA, at the time of the study. Joanne Stanraugh was Supervisor of the Brain Injury Rehabilitation Unit, Magee Rehabilitation Hospital, Philadelphia, PA, at the time of this study.

The authors wish to acknowledge Maureen Freda, Director of the Occupational Therapy Department at Magee Rehabilitation Hospital, for her assistance and encouragement.

have escalated. Among these efforts, much work has been done in the area of cognitive rehabilitation. Numerous computer and non-computerized protocols have been developed which are aimed at enhancing the reasoning and memory capacities of individuals with CHI. Currently, the focus of cognitive retraining is on the restoration of memory, perceptual, and reasoning skills which compose functional cognition. Only recently have the roles of metacognition and executive function been suggested as areas for investigation and intervention. As further study proceeds, executive function deficits are becoming increasingly recognized by rehabilitation professionals as major causes of dysfunction in individuals with CHI.

The article describes a research study which explored the nature of executive function deficits in individuals with CHI. A second aim of the study was to determine individual preference for cognitive retraining activity. The paper begins with a definition of and a brief review of the literature on executive function. The research, a multiple case design, is then presented. The paper concludes with suggestions for further research and intervention implications for individuals with executive function impairment.

DEFINITIONS AND LITERATURE REVIEW

Executive function is a category of cognition that fits into the meta-domain (or overseeing element) of human thought. Lezak (1982) suggests that initiation, flexibility, self monitoring, and cognitive organization are components of executive function. In other words, executive function is characterized not as the "*how*" of cognitive activity, but the "*if*" (Lezak, 1982). Without meta cognition, thought process does not occur.

Because of their vague nature, executive functions have only recently been the topic of theory and research. Methodologically, it is difficult to discriminate which components of cognition are responsible for the occurrence of an activity. For example, in the case where an individual is known to have frontal lobe damage, the inability to engage independently in a task could be a function of impairment in several arenas of cognition, only one of which is executive function.

One of the ways in which executive function can be investigated is through non-example. That is to say, if functional cognition is impaired, but standardized testing reveals no specific cognitive deficit, then executive function may be the suspect deficit.

In efforts to develop a standardized assessment of executive function, Lezak (1982) created the Tinker Toy Test (TTT) in which an individual is asked to construct an object from a selection of tinker toy pieces, to name it, and to make some comments regarding its use. During the administration of the test, no specific directions are given to the subject, thereby assessing the ability to plan, initiate, and think spontaneously. The instrument is scored on the number of pieces used, the complexity of construction itself, and the label for the construction. Other forms of assessment of executive function include observation of individuals engaged in activities which require initiation, choice, organization, and flexibility (Chelune and Moehle, in Imes, 1985).

Specific intervention strategies to mediate executive functional deficits have not been described in the literature. It seems as if executive function is subsumed under traditional remediation activities. However, a recent study (Johnson and Diller, 1983) pointed out the need to address executive function separately in treatment. The researchers noted that while right hemisphere stroke patients were able to improve their measured performance on a cognitive rehabilitation task, their ability to judge and subsequently regulate their own performance was impaired, leading to potential functional incapacity.

Because of recent recognition of the importance of the concept of executive function, few research studies have as yet been conducted to develop assessments or to investigate strategies to remediate deficits in executive function. However, the value of cognitive rehabilitation in general has been empirically supported. Therefore it is essential to investigate the role of executive functional deficits in functional cognitive impairment further and to develop effective assessment and intervention strategies to remediate these deficits. According to Parsons and Prigstano (1978), case study is a sound descriptive methodology for exploring the consequences of neuropathology and for testing the effects of intervention. The two case studies which follow are an attempt to characterize the different nature of executive function in each individual and to describe the approach to various methods of cognitive rehabilitation.

METHODOLOGY

A multiple case study design was used to describe executive function in persons with CHI and to determine the relationship among executive functional deficit, locus of control and preference of two different cognitive retraining modalities. All subjects were for CHI rehabilitation, suffered frontal lobe impairment, and were not receiving treatment for any other non-relating disorder. They were also screened for premorbid status to eliminate the possibility of pre-existing conditions which might be responsible for their performance in the study.

Each subject participated in the study for a period of three weeks. They were pre-tested for the initiation element of executive function, overall executive function, locus of control, degree of disability, and cognitive ability. To assess initiation and executive function the Tinker Toy Test and the Initiation Log, developed by the researchers (see Table 1) were used. The Rotter's I-E Scale was used to test locus of control and the Disability Rating Scale was used to assess overall level of disability. To ascertain cognitive function, a Rancho Score was assigned to each subject. Further patient information, including scores from standardized testing, medical evaluation, social evaluation, and progress, was gleaned from a qualitative review of progress notes. Locus of control and disability level were tested in order to determine if there was a change in these functions as the subjects participated in the cognitive activities.

Following pre-testing, each subject was observed in daily one hour sessions of occupational therapy as s/he participated in three weeks of structured cognitive retraining. During the first week of the study, subjects were assigned only to computerized cognitive retraining activities. During the second week, subjects were assigned to paper and pencil activities only. Subjects were permitted to choose between paper and pencil and computerized cognitive activities during the third week of study. These three methods were selected to determine the relationship between executive function

TABLE 1

INITIATION LOG

SCORING:

1 = independent initiation of the intended therapeutic activity without any cues from therapist
2 = initiation of activity with one verbal cue from therapist
3 = initiation of activity with more than one verbal cue which does not mention the modality
4 = more than one verbal cue give to direct the patient to the appropriate therapeutic modality
5 = no willingness to participate in activity unless coerced by the therapist
6 = refusal to do the therapeutic activity

CASE # ____________ DATE: ____________ COMPUTER OR PAPER/PENCIL

Therapeutic goals for therapy session:

Modality (be specific) ____

ACTIVITY	INITIATION FREQUENCY	LEVEL

Note any behaviors and verbailizations related to the therapeutic activity:

Scores or notation of patient performance: ____________________

____

____

deficit and activity preference. The Rotters I-E scale and the Tinker Toy Test were repeated following the first and second weeks of the study. Qualitative analysis and daily scoring of the initiation log were conducted throughout the study. Charts were also reviewed by the investigators following the termination of each patient's participation for qualitative trends regarding the subjects executive and cognitive functions.

The next section describes case study data and analysis of two subjects who participated in the study.

FINDINGS

Case Study #1 – John

John is a 21-year-old white male who sustained a closed head injury and paraplegia after a serious fall. Prior to his injury, John was a senior college student preparing for a career in agricultural finance. His accident occurred the night before he was to sit for a qualifying examination in his chosen career.

Upon admission to the emergency room (ER) at a local hospital, it was noted that the patient sustained multiple orthopedic injuries. Neurologically, the patient was comatose for two weeks, resulting from multiple brain injuries including a temporal contusion, a right subarachnoid hemorrhage, and a left basal pulmonary contusion. When admitted to the ER following the accident, the patient was given a Glascow Coma Rating of 9-10. The length of post traumatic amnesia was reported at 45 days.

The patient remained in the acute care hospital approximately two months during which orthopedic surgery and neurosurgery were performed to reduce and set fractures and to maintain normal intracranial pressure. John was discharged to an inpatient brain injury rehabilitation unit where he remained for a period of five months. He is currently receiving outpatient therapy on a daily basis while living with his father and two siblings. John is moderately neurologically disabled and is just beginning to ambulate with the assistance of crutches.

This case study was conducted over a period of three weeks during the patient's inpatient residency. On pre-testing John scored in the moderately disabled range (6) on the Disability Rating Scale (DRS) with a Rancho Rating of 7. He received 10 out of a maximum twelve points on the initial Tinker Toy Test. Initial Rotters I-E score was 10.

Table 2 depicts descriptive statistics for the repeated measures of the Rotters I-E and the Tinker Toy Test. Table 3 displays pre- and post-test scores on the DRS and the Rancho. Table 4 presents mean initiation scores on the initiation log for each of the three weeks of the study.

Observations and recordings of the subject's behavior during therapeutic sessions over the three week period reveal that John did not demonstrate a preference for either cognitive modality. Baseline testing indicated that John was able to engage in a scheduled activity once he entered the room where familiar equipment was present. However, following the termination of the activity, John had to be directed to the next activity. During the first week of the study,

TABLE 2

Rotter I-E and TTT Raw Scores

Case #	Rotter I-E			Tinker Toy		
	Pre	#1	#2	Pre	#1	#2
Case #1	10	11	10	10	9	8
Case #2	10	10	10	6	6	5

TABLE 3

DISABILITY RATING SCALE SCORES AND LEVELS OF COGNITIVE FUNCTION (RANCHO) SCORES: PRE- AND POST-TEST

CASE #	DRS		Rancho LOCF	
	Pre	Post	Pre	Post
Case #1	6	3	7	7
Case #2	8	4	7	7

TABLE 4

Mean Initiation Scores by Week for Each Phase of the Study

Case #	Pre-Test	Week One	Week Two	Week Three
Case #1	2.0	2.0	2.0	2.0
Case #2	4.0	1.6	2.2	1.0

John demonstrated similar and consistent behavior. He always asked for direction to an activity and was only able perform after he was told which task to undertake. Once directed to the computer, John was able to complete the demands of the task in front of him independently. However, any change in activity required further direction from the occupational therapist. The same initiation behavior was noted on the initiation log during week two. Over the course of ten days John received an initiation rating of 2 consistently. During week three John was unable to select the computer or the paper and pencil activity, even though he was familiar with both, and deferred to the occupational therapist for direction. Recordings of verbalization revealed that John was invested in the activity, once directed to it. For example, on day three of week one, during a computer task, the occupational therapist quoted John as saying, "I should be able to think and to see the word, like you did. That's what the game is all about." Similar verbalizations occurred throughout the three weeks regardless of the type of cognitive retraining activity.

Even after the activity became familiar and less challenging, John still would ask for, and follow, the direction of the therapist. For example, on day 5 of week one the subject said, "The words should get new, this is too easy. Does Gail (the occupational therapist) want me only to play these?"

Chart extraction revealed that John was able to perform within normal limits on proverb interpretation and on number recall tasks. However, progress notes continued to indicate a short term memory deficit and *concrete operational thought patterns*. Notes regarding affect described that patient as superficially aware of his disability and unwilling to make appropriate future plans consistent with the extent of his disability.

Scores on intermediate Rotter and TTT tests and post-tests did not reveal any significant change with one exception. Each administration of the Tinker Toy Test assessment revealed a decrease in score although the scores remained relatively high.

Preliminary Conclusions on Case #1

Initiation scores and qualitative data reveal that John was unable to initiate activity when presented with two or more options, even if both options were familiar to him. However, once directed to an activity, he was able to respond to its demands providing that the activity was familiar or structured. This initiation pattern became evident during week three of the case study. John was unable to select either cognitive modality on any of the days, but he was able to perform once the occupational therapist directed him to an activity.

It is not surprising that the scores on the Tinker Toy Test, particularly the pre-test administration, did not support the qualitative findings of impairment of executive function derived from the initiation log and chart notes. Because the patient was able to function after being directed to an activity, he was able to score well on the Tinker Toy Test in which the materials were presented to him in a structured space, with no option to engage in another task. Thus, John was able to perform successfully if instructed in what to do. Further investigation into why his scores decreased over the three week period is necessary to determine the cause.

This discrepancy between standardized and/or structured testing and daily performances was further supported by data obtained through chart extraction. Nursing, social service, medicine and therapy progress notes continuously reported a short term memory impairment, difficulty in initiation, and concrete reasoning during daily therapeutic, recreational, and self care activity. However, neurological testing revealed no specific cognitive impairments, as evidenced by John's ability to perform well on number recall tasks and to interpret proverbs using formal operational reasoning. It can, therefore, be suggested that John's functional deficits may be, in large part, caused by executive function impairment rather than impairment in specific information processing functions.

Further attention needs to be directed to John's adaptation to his disability and his willingness to engage in therapeutic activity. Chart extraction reveals John seems to be unrealistic about his future. He expects to walk without assistance and to resume his career plans. Additionally, there is no notation in the chart about John's affective change or concern over current or future status. Thus, he has a superficial grasp of his disability and his potential. These behaviors and patterns are furthur demonstrations of executive function deficit as defined. Included in the construct of executive function are the ability to be flexible in thinking, the capacity for self monitoring, and future planning capacity. John demonstrates impairment in each of these areas.

Case #2–Al

Al was a 39-year-old white male who was struck by an automobile while en route to his probation officer. Upon admission to the ER, Al was comatose and had multiple orthopedic and pulmonary complications. Length of coma and post traumatic amnesia upon regaining consciousness were not noted in the rehabilitation chart. The patient was treated for pulmonary, neurological, and orthopedic injuries and then transferred to an inpatient brain injury unit of an urban rehabilitation hospital approximately one month post-insult.

Upon admission, Al was reported to be inappropriate in social conversation. Although cooperative with hospital staff, he was preoccupied with his left lower extremity, which had been fractured during the accident. Nursing admission notes indicate that Al confabulated when he was unable to recall information. Cognitively, he demonstrated slow processing time, attentional deficits, and short term visual memory.

Subsequent progress notes from all disciplines confirmed that Al demonstrated impulsivity in his thought patterns, mood swings, remote memory deficits and variable recent memory. Executive functional deficits include difficulty with self-monitoring, poor insight and self appraisal, inflexibility in problem solving, and difficulty with initiating activity. He also demonstrated constructional apraxia.

Premorbidly, Al had been incarcerated for theft. He also had a long history of drug use. At the time of his accident, Al was on probation, lived with his wife and 13-year-old child, and was unemployed. While he had initially planned to return home following discharge from the rehabilitation hospital, he eventually decided to live with his mother, where the environment was less challenging.

At the initiation of the study, Al had DR score of 8, which placed him in the moderately severe range of disability, and a Rancho Score of 7. Rotter's I-E score was 10, indicating that he perceived himself as neither internally or externally controlled. TTT score was 6 due to Al's inability to construct complex objects or name his simple construction. Mean pre-test initiation score was 4.0 during occupational therapy sessions, indicating that the subject needed extensive cueing to select and attend to an activity.

During the first week of the study, Al was able to initiate activity after becoming familiar with the computer. (See Table 4 for initiation scores.) However, once frustrated or overchallenged, Al required cueing to return to task. Qualitative data indicate that Al showed a preference for computer activity in which he felt competent. He selected software with which he was familiar and which he had already mastered.

The subject demonstrated similar patterns during week two of the study. He initiated action when the activity was predetermined or familiar. During week three, he demonstrated a clear preference for the computer. Al stated "I love it," when referring to the computer. When asked why, he indicated that he benefited from the immediate feedback and felt competent. However, the therapist/observer noted that even though Al felt competent, he was not performing accurately and was unable to monitor or evaluate his own performance realistically.

Data from chart extraction were consistent with Al's performance in the study. Although distractable, he was able to perform tasks in a structured environment if they were familiar, not challenging and did not require new learning. When unable to complete a task, the subject would cease activity and become angry. Once experiencing failure, Al required cueing in order to return to productivity. Further, his insight and self appraisal remained compromised. Over the course of the study, confabulation decreased as the subject's short term memory improved.

Preliminary Conclusions #2

Al's behavioral patterns revealed that while able to initiate familiar activity, any distraction obstructed his ability to perform purposeful action. Furthermore, Al demonstrated executive functional deficits in the area of self monitoring, inflexibility of thought, and insight. It is not surprising that Al showed a preference for the computer over other types of activity when considering the structured nature of computerized activity. In addition, the computer provided immediate feedback, positive feedback and frequent cueing.

Al's poor performance on the TTT was not only compromised by his constructional apraxia but also by his inability to judge his own limitations and explain his behavior in light of them. Al's premorbid function seemed exaggerated in his rehabilitation efforts. Data from chart extraction support that Al did and does not demonstrate awareness of how his lack of control impairs his ability to function. Therefore, Al seems to function well on the portions of standardized assessments which present little challenge, but he is unable to demonstrate skill competence, since poor performance may be a result of poor self monitoring rather than absence of skill.

IMPLICATIONS

From case studies and the literature on executive function, several implications arise regarding the assessment and treatment of closed head injury.

First, it is clear that executive function needs to be addressed both in assessment and treatment of individuals who have sustained frontal lobe damage. It is becoming increasingly recognized that executive function impairment can be more devastating than impairment in other arenas of cognition and may prevent efficient use of remaining cognitive and functional skills. Each of the case studies demonstrates a unique constellation of executive function deficits which results in extremely different clinical pictures. Additionally, the interaction of premorbid factors, other function and clinical sequelae and executive function needs to be assessed in order to obtain an accurate clinical and functional picture of each individual.

Second, the case studies suggest complimentarity of formal and informal assessment. Individuals with executive function impairments do perform differently on structured tasks, thereby potentially masking or exaggerating deficits. For example, in Case #1, John performed better on structured tasks once directed to them, than on similar tasks in an undirected field setting. In contrast, Al performed worse on standardized tests than on similar tasks in a natural environment, due to his incapacity to tolerate frustration and modify his behavior accordingly. It follows that from the case studies that rehabilitation professionals should rely on assessment measures which combine formal measures with qualitative data such as observation and recorded professional impressions.

A third and most important implication is for treatment. While executive function may improve with neurological recovery, it has been documented as one of the most frequent residual deficits in CHI. Therefore, traditional rehabilitation strategies which focus on training a patient in compensatory strategies may be insufficient to promote function, if one is unable to initiate or use strategies in an organized fashion. Intervention which combines compensation with environmental adaption may be more effective promoting function than skill training by itself. In other words, intervention with individuals who exhibit executive functional deficits should focus both on the individual and on the environment.

Finally, findings from the case studies suggest implications for research methodology investigating closed head injury. It seems that integration of research methods is most effective strategy for exploring the breadth and depth of closed head injury incidence, characterization assessment, and intervention. As demonstrated in the case studies, data from formal, structured measures seemed to reveal only what subjects were capable of doing in structured settings. Formal testing did not demonstrate the effect of executive functional deficits on function in undirected daily activity. Therefore, it is not unreasonable that formal measures in scientific investigation will neglect the same evidence omitted from formal measures in the case studies. Researchers should therefore consider hybrid methodology as a strategy for investigating closed head injury function and treatment.

REFERENCES

Chelune, G.J. and Moehle, K.A. in Imes C. (1985). Cognitive rehabilitation of brain-damaged patients: An annotated bibliography. *Cognitive Rehabilitation*, *3* (3):8-19.

Johnson, C.W. and Diller, L. (1983). Error evaluation ability of right hemisphere brain-lesioned patients who have had perceptual cognitive retraining. *Journal of Clinical Neuropsychology*, *5* (4):401-2.

Lezak, M. (1982). The problem of assessing executive functions. *International Journal of Psychology*, *17*:281-297.

Parsons, O.A. and Prigatano, G.P. (1978). Methodological considerations in neuropsychological research. *Journal of Consulting and Clinical Psychology*, *46* (4):608-619.

Professional Staff of Rancho Los Amigos Hospital (1977). *Levels of Cognitive Function*. Downey, CA, Rancho Los Amigos Hospital.

Rotter, J. (1966). Generalized expectancy for internal versus external control of reinforcement. *Psychological Monographs*, 80:1-28.

Stroke Clients' Perceptions of Disability and Treatment

Lyn Jongbloed, PhD, OT(C)
Debra Morgan, BSR

SUMMARY. Twenty subjects who had experienced a stroke and were serving as a control group in a larger research project, were interviewed regarding the effect the stroke had had on their lives and their perceptions of the occupational therapy they had received. The majority of the subjects had very little understanding of the nature of a stroke but were well able to articulate the effect the stroke had had on their lives. How each person experienced a stroke was very different, yet the losses each felt related to North American values of independence, mobility, individual control and coping. Treatment received in occupational therapy was most commonly described in terms of games; very few people had grasped the notion that the central purpose of occupational therapy was to help them to perform daily living tasks independently. Therapists should consequently consider the use of more functionally oriented treatment.

INTRODUCTION

Health professionals and people with disabilities differ in the way in which they view disability. Health professionals treat diseases, i.e., abnormalities in the structure and function of body organs and

---

Lyn Jongbloed is Associate Professor, School of Rehabilitation Medicine, T106—Third Floor, ACU, 2211 Wesbrook Mall, Vancouver, B.C. V6T 1W5, Canada. The National Health Research and Development Program (NHRDP) funded the study from which this data set is drawn.

The authors acknowledge the contributions of Jan Gauthier, Johanne Morin, Alix McGinity, Gloria Altman, Ann Cooper, Cara Shorter and Cathy Brighton to data collection and analysis. They are also thankful for the support received from directors of three Occupational Therapy Departments: Brenda Robinson (Holy Family Hospital), Bridget Duckworth (G.F. Strong Rehabilitation Centre) and Dawn Daechsel (Lions Gate Hospital).

systems (Eisenberg, 1977). They are concerned with providing objective, scientific accounts of illness that are devoid of cultural meaning. Thus, they describe a stroke as a cerebrovascular accident, as a result of which the person may be paralyzed or weak on the side of the body opposite to the site of the stroke. Neurological deficits of all kinds may occur in addition to the motor signs. Patients, on the other hand, suffer illnesses; they experience changes in states of being and social function (Eisenberg, 1977). They are concerned with the human experience of the disability and struggle to understand what it means to them. They employ explanatory models to construct and interpret what has happened to them (Kleinman, 1978). Psychological, social and cultural factors influence the way individuals experience disability and how they interpret symptoms and evaluate treatment (Good & Good, 1980).

While much is known about the biological correlates of a stroke, relatively little is known about the way in which people who have had a stroke explain what has happened to them, or how they understand and experience the treatment they receive. The objectives of this research were to gain some understanding of how people experienced the effects of a stroke and to examine how they perceived the occupational therapy they received in hospital.

METHOD

This research was a subsection of a larger research project, the objective of which was to determine the effectiveness of a leisure skills training program with stroke survivors. In the larger research project, the 20 individuals assigned to the experimental group received occupational therapy intervention which was aimed at assisting them to resume former leisure activities and/or learn to engage in new activities. The 20 individuals assigned to the control group did not receive occupational therapy intervention, but spent five one-hour sessions talking to an occupational therapist. During this time, the therapist had an opportunity to explore what the stroke meant to these clients and how they viewed the treatment they had received. Interviews took place in the clients' homes.

The data for the research reported here were drawn from interviews with the 20 individuals who formed the control group in the larger study. All subjects had incurred a stroke within the past 12 months, had completed a rehabilitation program, and were not severely aphasic (i.e., could follow a one-step command and had some means of self expression, e.g., gesture, verbal expression or communication aid). Eight subjects had incurred a right CVA and 12 a left CVA; 13 were males and 7 were females. The mean age was 69.6 years, and ages ranged from 42 to 86 years.

A semi-structured interview guide was used to direct the content of the interviews. Questions focused on clients' explanatory models, i.e., how they explained what had happened to them and their perceptions of treatment (see Table 1). Questions were not necessarily phrased or asked in the order listed in Table 1.

RESULTS

Explanatory Models

Table 2 summarizes subjects' responses to questions about the stroke. The majority of individuals did not know what had caused their stroke. Several exhibited knowledge of the contributing factors of stress and a diet high in fat and/or cholesterol. One individual expressed his thoughts about diet and stress-related factors this way: "There might be an artery that is blocked. I'm very careful with my diet. I eat only two eggs a week. I don't know enough about stroke to avoid it, but I don't eat a lot of junk food. In other words, I should not have a stroke because I'm careful with what I eat, and I wasn't worked to death." Another who mentioned diet said the cause was "Too much ketchup, too much peanut butter, too much oil."

The majority did not know why the stroke had occurred when it did and did not know how the stroke worked. Examples of responses which indicated the best understanding were these. "A platelet broke away and it flowed along 'til it got to a small artery and couldn't pass through, so my arm and leg like died." "There's a clot on the brain on one side and so the paralysis is on the right. They usually come in threes. You get two light ones and then a heavy one and then you can get another one anytime and my doctor says they're usually on the other side." "I think it starts up here in

Table 1

Interview Guide

Explanatory Models

1. What do you think caused your stroke?
2. Why do you think you had the stroke when you did?
3. How does the stroke work?
4. How severe is your stroke? Do you think it will have a long or a short course?
5. What do you think the stroke does to you?
6. What are the chief problems the stroke has caused for you?
7. What do you fear most about your stroke?

(Kleinman, Eisenberg & Good, 1978)

Perceived Value of Treatment

1. What sort of treatment did you receive in hospital?
2. In what way did the treatment help you?
3. What sort of treatment did the occupational therapist give you?
4. Which of the occupational therapy activities did you find most helpful?
5. Which occupational therapy activities did you find least helpful?
6. Have you maintained the level of function you had in hospital?

the brain. And I think the blood from the burst vessel seeps into your body and you lose control of your limbs and your voice; and it's a terrible feeling, you know."

Eleven of the subjects expressed the opinion that they had had a mild stroke. Eight subjects thought their stroke was of medium severity; they had seen people who were both better and worse off.

Table 2

Summary of Responses - Explanatory Models

Cause of Stroke	
Do not know	13
Stress	2
Diet	2
High blood pressure	1
Prescribed medication	1
Smoking	1
What the stroke does	
Affects arm and leg	6
Inability to do activities	5
Poor memory/concentration	2
Poor speech	2
Loss of interest	1
Fatigue	1
Feel useless	1
Why the stroke occurred when it did	
Do not know	16
Stress	2
High blood pressure	2
Chief problems caused by stroke	
Loss of function in arm and/or leg	5
Inactivity/boredom	5
Curtailment of physical activities	3
Not being able to drive	2
Poor memory	1
Poor speech	1
Inability to read	1
Rolelessness	1
How the stroke works	
Do not know	14
Affects brain	3
Restriction of blood vessel	3
Severity of Stroke	
Mild	11
Moderate	8
Severe	1
Fears	
Recurrence of stroke	7
Not much improvement	4
Dependence	3
Falling	2
Not being wanted	1
Death	1
Nothing	2

N = 20

Many said they thought the stroke would affect them for the rest of their lives.

When asked what the stroke does, several subjects mentioned reduced function in the affected arm and leg. One man expressed it this way: "I can't talk properly and my hand and leg don't work properly." Others talked about the activities they could no longer do. "I can't knit or crochet any more. I can't write. I had to go to the bank and change my signature." Another said, "Well, it set me back quite a bit; like yesterday, I managed to peel those pears, but it was no picnic. I'm right handed and have no strength in it." Some focused on how it made them feel. For example, "It eliminates me from so much, you know. The interest just isn't there anymore for all the things I used to do." Another said, "I'm useless. I can't do anything."

In terms of the chief problems the stroke had caused, the most common answers were (1) loss of function in the arm and leg, and (2) inactivity/boredom. A few subjects talked about the curtailment of social activities such as curling, lawn bowling and golf, and others mentioned the inability to drive. A woman whose husband had hired a housekeeper since her stroke expressed her sense of loss this way, "Everyone can get along without me. My housekeeper and my daughter make all the decisions." Patients with relatively similar functional levels often gave very different answers to the question of the chief problem caused by the stroke. The problem or loss that was most significant to an individual was determined chiefly by his/her age, value system and previous life style.

In terms of fears about the stroke, fear of another stroke was mentioned most frequently. Other mentioned fears were falling, dependence, death, not being wanted and not improving. A few subjects said they feared nothing.

Therapy

Responses to questions about therapy are summarized in Table 3. The majority of individuals identified having received treatment from occupational and physical therapists; some mentioned speech therapy. When asked what treatment had helped them, the majority were unable to specify a particular treatment that had been benefi-

Table 3

Summary of Responses - Therapy

Treatment perceived as beneficial	
Unable to specify	12
Muscle stimulator	3
No treatment helpful	3
Ultrasound	1
Exercises	1
Treatment received in O.T.	
Games	18
Dressing	1
Meal preparation	1
O.T. activities perceived as most helpful	
Unable to specify	16
Relationship with therapist	2
Sandbags	1
Dressing	1
O.T. activities perceived as least helpful	
Unable to specify	16
Puzzles	3
Baking	1
Level of function since discharge	
Doing more	18
Doing less	2

cial. Three subjects mentioned the muscle stimulator; one phrased his belief in this treatment this way: "The muscle stimulator really pulled the muscles inside, and I think if they had just had more of that, they would have started to work on their own." Ultrasound was perceived as helpful by one person, and exercises by another. Three people said the therapists did not do much good.

When asked what treatment the occupational therapist had given them, subjects mostly described activities they had done and games they had played. Examples included some of the following responses: "Pushing a balloon back and forth using my left hand." "They had a blue bench in front of me, and I had to slide the bean bags and pick them up. We'd get hockey sticks and we had to shove the bean bag across to the person with the stick." "She had a board with lights, and you have to tell her how many I miss on the left." One person mentioned dressing and another, meal preparation.

Some misunderstood the goal of certain interventions. For example, one person thought a test of perceptual function was a form of treatment for his hand. "These two fingers are stiff. When I hold something it falls off, so they gave me this little box with different designs. She put it in my hand and asked me to close my hand and point to the design on the card that was drawn on my hand."

Most subjects were unable to specify which occupational therapy activities had been the most helpful. One mentioned dressing, another sandbags. Two subjects said the relationship with the therapist was the most important aspect of treatment. One of the subjects expressed it this way, "The O.T. was very helpful. She was a friend, too. I could talk to her. She got me up and moving when I didn't really want to." Activities perceived as least helpful included puzzles and baking.

When asked whether they had maintained the level of function they had in hospital, the majority noted they had improved. However, one individual said, "I don't do everything I used to do in hospital because my wife says it's easier if she does it for me." In another case the spouse said, "I can't ever get her to do the things they told me she could do while in hospital. She just says she can't do anything with one hand, so I should do it for her now, and when her hand gets better she'll start to do it for herself."

DISCUSSION

Subjects' understanding of the nature of a stroke and their explanations of the cause of this event were heterogeneous. For the most part, they did not have a good understanding of these issues. It is quite likely that these people had been given adequate medical explanations but that they could not incorporate such explanations into their own belief systems regarding how their bodies functioned. Their explanations likely resulted from a complicated process of incorporating some ideas and rejecting others. The implication of this finding is that health professionals should provide such education and explanations on several different occasions.

Although they were not clear what a stroke was, these people had no difficulty describing the effect the stroke had had on their everyday lives. A stroke reduces the efficiency of a most basic resource, one's body. What these people experienced was an inability to use parts of their body efficiently. They consequently viewed the difficulties in living which resulted from the stroke as constituting the entire disorder. What the stroke meant to them was a loss of function; the nature and causes of a stroke were not important to them.

According to Lipowski (1969) illness has one of four psychological meanings – threat, loss, no significance and gain. Both loss and threat emerged as strong themes. The loss of body functions and of personally significant roles was painful for many of these people. What each individual experienced as his/her chief loss was influenced by his/her age, value system and lifestyle. The possibilities of another stroke and of dependence were feared by many.

There were considerable differences among individuals in terms of what treatment they considered helpful. Some thought that treatment *applied to them* was most beneficial. Others recognized the importance of active involvement in regaining strength and control in the affected limb. Occupational therapists could spend more time attempting to understand what the stroke means to that particular patient and eliciting more information regarding treatment he/she expects will be helpful.

Most individuals described the treatment they received in occupational therapy in terms of games. Noticeably absent from their accounts of occupational therapy was the notion that the primary goal of treatment is to increase the individual's ability to perform tasks independently. If clients who have received occupational therapy are going to be effective advocates of our profession, it is important that they understand the goals of treatment. Since it appears that people remember the activity rather than the goals of the activity, occupational therapists would do well to make treatment programs more functionally oriented, particularly since research has not been able to identify any differences in outcome between stroke patients who receive sensorimotor integrative treatment and those who receive functional treatment (Jongbloed, Stacey & Brighton, 1989).

CONCLUSION

Explanatory models were elicited from 20 people who had incurred a stroke within the last 12 months. Illness reality, the person's interpretation of symptoms, is both a personal and social reality grounded in what is of importance to that individual, and is linked to sociocultural beliefs and values. Each of these people experienced their stroke very differently, yet the losses they felt and feared relate to North American values of independence, mobility, individual control and coping. Therapists could enhance both the quality of their treatment, and their clients' perceptions of the value of that treatment by spending more time eliciting the web of meanings in terms of which their clients experience disability and evaluate treatment.

Most subjects described the occupational therapy they received in terms of games, and had not realized that the chief purpose of this therapy was to assist them to perform daily living tasks independently. Therapists should consequently consider the use of more functionally-oriented treatment.

REFERENCES

Eisenberg, L. (1977). Disease & illness: distinctions between professional and popular ideas of sickness. *Culture, Medicine & Psychiatry, 1*: 9-23.

Good, B.J., Good, M.D. (1980). The meanings of symptoms: a cultural hermeneutic model for clinical practice. In Eisenberg, L. and Kleinman, A. (Eds). *The Relevance of Social Science for Medicine*. D. Reidel Pub Co, Boston.

Jongbloed, L., Stacey, S., Brighton, C. (1989). Stroke rehabilitation: Sensorimotor integrative treatment versus functional treatment. *American Journal of Occupational Therapy*, *43*, (6), 391-397.

Kleinman, A. (1978). Problems and prospects in comparative cross-cultural medical and psychiatric studies. In Kleinman, A., Kunstadter, P., Alexander, E.R., Gate, J.L. (Eds). *Culture and Healing in Asian Societies*. Schenkman Publishing Co., Cambridge, Mass.

Kleinman, A, Eisenberg, L. Good, B. (1978). Culture, illness and care: clinical lessons from anthropologic and cross-cultural research. *Annals of Internal Medicine, 33*, (2), 251-258.

Lipowski, Z.J. (1969). Psychosocial aspects of disease. *Annals of Internal Medicine*, *71*: 1197-1206.

SOMETHING NEW AND DIFFERENT

OTDBASE: An Occupational Therapy Literature Search Service

Marilyn Ernest, MA, OT(C)

SUMMARY. This article describes the rationale behind the development of an "only occupational therapy" computerized literature search service. OTDBASE, the clinically-oriented index and data base, contains all relevant information about all articles from eight occupational therapy (OT) journals from 1970 to the present and includes up to 10 lines of abstract per article. The service was developed for purposes of contributing to continuing education and research efforts in occupational therapy.

INTRODUCTION

The purpose of this article is to describe the rationale behind the development of a new literature search service for occupational therapists and to explain both why and how it can be used by clinicians, students and researchers.

Marilyn Ernest is Associate Professor, Department of Occupational Therapy, The University of Western Ontario, London, Ontario, Canada N6A 3K7. Her mailing address is 1778 Attawandaron Road London, Ontario, Canada, N6G 3N1.

Background

The development of an "only occupational therapy literature" computerized database search service (OTDBASE) grew out of the developer's long-term interest in the use of occupational therapy (OT) literature for purposes of continuing education and research. An early study (Ernest, Burton, & Keenleyside, 1978) described how the use of literature could lead to researchable questions and answers. A second study examined the use of the *Canadian Journal of Occupational Therapy* (*CJOT*) as reference material by authors published in *CJOT* over a 15 year period (Ernest, 1983). One conclusion reached was that very few *CJOT* authors were using this source of professional literature as a resource. This led to another concern as to whether or not clinicians, educators and students were able to make the fullest possible use of the increasing number of professional journals for purposes of continuing education and research. Accessibility to both professional journals and specific articles of concern to clinicians in the various journals was examined.

Accessibility

Occupational therapy literature can be found in many index and abstract systems. For example, when all eight occupational therapy journals in OTDBASE were examined, it was found that they were accessible in a total of 42 different indexing or abstracting services (see Table 1). It was also noted that the only service that contained all eight journals was OTDBASE.

It was felt by this author that clinicians, educators and students looking for specific occupational therapy information for continuing education or research purposes must: (a) have convenient access to these index and abstract systems; (b) have knowledge of each system in terms of the type of literature found in each system, or pay to have searches carried out in many systems; (c) be very wise at guessing the precise content of an article if no abstract is included in the printout; and (d) be accepting of the fact that computerized indexing and abstracting of occupational therapy literature has been carried out for a relatively few years, and therefore, literature relevant to one's area of interest could be missed. As well, it was im-

TABLE 1. Indexing and Abstracting Services

Indices/Abstracts	Occupational Therapy Journals							
	AJOT	AOTJ	CJOT	OTHC	OTJR	OTMH	POTG	POTP
Abstract of Health Care Management Studies						x		
Abstracts of Res. in Pastoral Care & Couns.						x	x	
Adolescent Mental Health Abstracts						x		
Australian Med. Index		x						
Behavioural Abstracts						x		
Bibliographic Index of Health Educ. Period.							x	
Biological Abstracts						x	x	
Bulletin Signaletique						x	x	
Cambridge Scientific Abstracts				x			x	
Chicago Psychoanalytic Literature Abstracts						x		
Child Development Abstracts & Bibliog.						x		
CIJE (Current Index to Journals in Education)					x			
CLOA (Current Index on Aging)				x			x	
Cumulative Indexing to Nursing and Allied Health Literature	x		x	x			x	x
Current Contents/Health Services Administ.								
Current Contents/Social & Behav. Sciences					x			
Current Lit. on Aging				x			x	
Exceptional Child Education Resources	x							
Excerpta Medica	x				x	x	x	x
Family Res. Database				x			x	x
Gerontology Abstracts							x	
Hospital Abstracts				x				
Hospital Lit.Index	x		x					
Index Medicus	x							
Index to Periodical Lit. on Aging				x			x	
Institute for Scientific Info.	x							
Internat. Journal of Rehab. Literature						x	x	x
Internat. Nursing Index							x	
Medical Abstracts Jour.						x		
Medical Care Review							x	
Medline	x							
O.T. Journal of Research				x		x	x	x
OTDBASE	x	x	x	x	x	x	x	x
Psychological Abstracts	x				x	x	x	x
Pschological Reader's Guide								x
Public Affairs Info. Bulletin							x	
Rehabilitation Literature	x					x	x	x
Rehab. & Phys. Medicine/ Gerontology/Geriatrics							x	
Sage Family Studies Abst.								x
Social Sciences Citation Index					x			
Social Work Research and Abstracts						x	x	
Sociology Abstracts							x	

portant to consider that once a searcher had found numerous articles of interest in the occupational therapy literature, the references in those articles could lead the searcher to further valuable primary reference sources in both occupational therapy and related fields.

DEVELOPMENT OF OTDBASE

OTDBASE, an "only occupational therapy" literature search service, was developed to fulfill a number of assumed needs, with practicing clinicians being the initial target of concern. The first assumption was that therapists working outside of university communities might have difficulty obtaining access to the numerous index and abstract systems and subsequently could be deterred from even trying to do so. The second assumption was that most occupational therapy departments in North America probably have access to at least two of the eight journals primarily written for occupational therapists, e.g., *American Journal of Occupational Therapy* (*AJOT*), *Occupational Therapy Journal of Research* (*OTJR*), *Canadian Journal of Occupational Therapy* (*CJOT*), *Occupational Therapy in Mental Health* (*OTMH*), *Occupational Therapy in Health Care* (*OTHC*), *Physical and Occupational Therapy in Geriatrics* (*POTG*), *Physical and Occupational Therapy in Pediatrics* (*POTP*), and *Australian Occupational Therapy Journal* (*AOTJ*). A third assumption was that an occupational therapy index should be developed that clearly (using clinical terminology) identified specific areas of practice concerns and let the recipient of such an indexed printout be aware of the availability, existence and relevance of other major occupational therapy literature sources.

OTDBASE INDEX

The OTDBASE index was developed by one occupational therapist (author) whose clinical experience includes practice in the areas of mental health, adult physical dysfunction and pediatrics, and teaching experience includes occupational therapy history, development and philosophy, orthotics and prosthetics, fieldwork, community and geriatric occupational therapy. The index is updated monthly.

The OTDBASE index (see Table 2) contains all articles in the eight occupational therapy journals from 1970 to the present. Printouts contain titles, subject and topic areas, first author, journal name, volume, number and year, and up to 10 lines of the complete or edited abstract. Many articles without abstracts have descriptive paragraphs taken from the article and used as abstracts. All articles are cross-referenced up to 6 times to ensure that relevant articles will not be missed by even a simple topic search.

A final assumption was that although journals may be available to the individual therapist, few practicing therapists can afford the *time* needed to search through years of back issues to find one or more articles of immediate concern to their patient care or research. Consequently the author believed that a reliable mail search service could alleviate this time problem and OTDBASE was developed in 1986.

OTDBASE SERVICE

The cost of OTDBASE searches has been kept modest to encourage its use, especially by therapists whose departmental budgets do not provide for such services. The costs range from $6.80 (US) for searches and printouts of all eight journal's articles relating to any three topics within any one subject area, to $42.50 (US) for all pediatric printouts. Pamphlets describing the service, the index and costs are available from the author. All search orders are normally filled within 72 hours and are returned by first class mail within the United States and Canada at no extra charge. Telephone orders are filled within 24 hours.

In conclusion, it was felt that by bringing all articles printed between 1970 and the present from the eight major journals devoted to occupational therapy into one search service (OTDBASE), and by making its use as easy and accessible as possible, a contribution has been made to continuing education and research in occupational therapy.

TABLE 2. OTDBASE Index

SUBJECT	TOPICS
Activity	Analysis: Crafts: Motivation: Research: Selection:
*ADL	Arch. Barriers: Chairs: Clothing: Cushions: Driving: Feeding: Programs: Wheelchairs: Aids:
AGED	Activity: Assessment: Chronic Care: Day Care: Function: Home Care: Motivation: Self Care: Research: Theory:
AMPUTEES	Aids: Myoelectric: Prosthesis: Rehab: Training:
ANATOMY	Anatomy: Neuroanatomy:
COMMUNITY	Cultural Influences: Private Practice: Programs:
*CVA	Apraxia: Evaluation: Groups: Perception:
FIELDWORK	Education: Evaluation: Objectives: Practice: Supervision:
HAND	Data Norms: Evaluation: Function: Sensation:
INSTRUMENTS	Development: Reliability: Standardization: Validation:
*LD	Auditory: Apraxia: Motor Control: Programs: PRN: Research: Screening: SI: Vestibular:
*MH	Activity: Acute: Addiction: Aged/A&RD: Body Image: Anorexia-Bulimia: B. Mod: Body Language: Children: Chronic Care: Community: Day Care: Evaluation: Forensic: Groups: Home Care: JD: SI: Phobia: Reorientation: Research: Theory: Voc. Rehab:
*MR	Activity: Adult: Assessment: Function: Theory: Programs: Research: Self Injury: Sensory: Vestibular Stimulation:
ORTHOTICS	Arm: Burns: Elbow: Hand: Leg: Materials: Neck: Quad: RA: Renal: Spasticity: Wrist:
OT as a Profession	Attitudes: Consultant: Ethics: Theory: Industry: History: Health Care: Roles: Manpower: Philosophy: Models: Law: Politics: Prof. Issues: Exam: Unions:
*OT Admin.	Management: Quality Assurance: Skills: Stats:
OT Education	Curriculum: Faculty: Research: Prof. Issues: Student Selection: Theory: Cont: Grad: U-Grad:
OT Practice	Art: Aquatics: Biofeedback: B.Mod: Community: Drama: Group: Horticulture: Music: Pain: Pets: Projectives: Poetry: Puppetry: Relaxation: Sex Counseling: Video:
OT Research	Clinical: Methods: Single Case: Statistics: Survey: Theory:
OT Teaching	Methods: Research:
	Abuse: Aids: Arthrogryposis: Assessment: Autism: Attitudes: Blind: Camping: Cancer: CDH: CP: RA:

TABLE 2 (continued)

Pediatrics	Communication: Community: Development: Feeding: Evaluation: Function: Hyperactivity: Incest: LD: Motor Control: OT and Parents: Infant: Prenatal: Instruments: Play: Rubella: Stimulation: Research: Sex Education: OT in School: Spina Bifida: Theory:
Physical Conditions	ALS: Aphasia: Arm: Back: Blind: Brain Damage: Hip: Burns: Cancer: Cardiac: COLD: CVA: Hand: Diabetes: Dying Pt./AIDS: Dysphagia: Evaluation: Finger: Function: Leg: OA: Parkinson: RA: Renal: Research: Shoulder: Spinal Cord: Stress: Wrist: MS: Pain:
*SI	Adults: Apraxia: Autism: History: Incidence: LD: Language: MH: Motor Control: Programs: PRN: Reflex: Research: Tactile: Theory: Vest. Stim:
Technical Devices	ADL: Communication: Computer: Electronics: Video: Vision:
Vocational	Assessment: Automation: Counseling: Leisure: Role: Retirement: Prevoc: Rehab: Tools: Work:

*Abbreviation Definitions-
- ADL- Activities of Daily Living
- CVA- Cerebral Vascular Accident (Stroke)
- LD- Learning Disabilities
- MH- Mental Health
- MR- Mental Retardation
- OT Admin.- Occupational Therapy Administration
- SI- Sensory Integration

REFERENCES

Ernest, M., Burton, H., & Keenleyside, J. (1978). The literature review: an integral part of the research process. *Canadian Journal of Occupational Therapy, 45*, 107-109.

Ernest, M. (1983). Canadian Journal of Occupational Therapy: A Reflection of Professional Growth. *Canadian Journal of Occupational Therapy, 50*, 165-169.

BOOK REVIEW

WHY CAN'T SHARON KOWALSKI COME HOME? Karen Thompson and Julie Andrzejewski. *San Francisco, CA: Spinsters/ Aunt Lute Book Company, P.O. Box 410687, San Francisco, CA 94141, 1988, 227 pages plus two appendices.*

Why Can't Sharon Kowalski Come Home? is a profoundly important book for all occupational therapists regardless of clinical specialty or professional role. While substantiating many basic beliefs associated with occupational therapy, the book's central thesis is that societal prejudice and intolerance, as expressed through individual action, can be used to violate a person's fundamental rights. Powerfully exposed is the degree to which handicappism, sexism, and heterosexism (the belief that heterosexism is superior to homosexuality and thus the only acceptable sexual preference), pervade our collective thinking and justify paternalistic repudiation of a disabled individual's self-determination. Through a provocative analysis of our legal and health care systems, *Why Can't Sharon Kowalski Come Home*? asks us to confront our biases and their potential interference with quality of care.

This book recounts the events which occurred to Sharon Kowalski, a lesbian women who suffered a severe head injury in 1983 when her car was hit by a drunk driver. At the time of the accident and for four years prior, Sharon Kowalski and Karen Thompson had lived together in a lesbian marriage, known only to their closest friends. Almost immediately following the accident, Donald Kowalski, Sharon's father, attempted to exclude Karen Thompson from his daughter's life. Hoping to convince him of the importance of her continued involvement in Sharon's recovery, Karen informed him of their relationship. This information provoked Donald Kowalski instead to attempt to prohibit Karen's visits through a series of legal maneuvers. Incounter action, Karen Thompson filed for legal guardianship. Strong documentation (some of which was provided by occupational therapists) substantiated the therapeutic benefits of Karen's daily involvement in Sharon's care, as well as Sharon's consistently expressed desire to return to her home with Karen. Nonetheless, Donald Kowalski was awarded, and Karen Thompson was denied, guardianship.

A succession of further legal judgements gave Donald Kowalski authority to deny visitations from Karen Thompson, Sharon's former friends, and Sharon's legal advocates. In July of 1985, Sharon was moved to a nursing facility close to her parent's home which lacked adequate rehabilitation services. Although the courts had mandated competency assessments every six months, no assessments occurred from the date of that move through July of 1988 when the book went to press.

Why Can't Sharon Kowalski Come Home? is a painful book to read. In great detail, the book describes actions by "professionals" which emanated from personal bigotry and ultimately deprived Sharon Kowalski of not only her right to self-determination, but of appropriate rehabilitation services as well. In her struggle, Karen Thompson progressively sees that Sharon Kowalski's rights were expunged precisely because she was a lesbian and an "unmarried" women and a person with a severe disability.

The implications of this book for occupational therapists are many. Fundamentally, it is a case study which evokes deserved pride in our longstanding professional beliefs. To name but two examples: our belief in an individual's right to self-determination, regardless of the extent of disability; and our belief in addressing capacity and health well beyond a myopic fascination with incapacity and pathology.

Beyond a comforting support of our beliefs, however, *Why Can't Sharon Kowalski Come Home?* challenges us. Tragically, Sharon Kowalski's story is not unique. Her story is the story of countless others who live in our nursing homes, who live on our streets, or who live with AIDS (to name but a few examples). It is the story of those who are too disabled to be advocates for themselves and yet are dependent upon a health care system which metes out its limited resources in an uneven and prejudicial manner. The stories of these people painfully reveal that advocacy against handicappism, however vital, is insufficient unto itself. *Why Can't Sharon Kowalski Come Home?* challenges its readers to name and render obsolete other societal "isms" which, as powerfully as handicappism, serve to devalue and then discard certain persons. This is an ethical challenge which has always been inherent in the practice of good occupational therapy everywhere.

Wendy Wood, MA, OTR/L